Instructor's Manual to Accompany

Community Health Nursing

CONCEPTS AND PRACTICE

FIFTH EDITION

Judith Ann Allender, RN,C, MSN, EdD
Professor
Department of Nursing
College of Health and Human Services
California State University
Fresno, California

Barbara Walton Spradley, RN, MN
Associate Professor Emeritus
School of Public Health
University of Minnesota
Minneapolis, Minnesota

Prepared by
Judith Ann Allender, RN,C, MSN, EdD

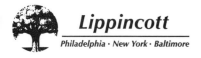
Lippincott
Philadelphia · New York · Baltimore

Ancillary Editor   Doris S. Wray
Compositor: LWW
Printer/Binder: Victor

ISBN: 0-7817-2957-2

Any procedure or practice described in this book should be applied by the health care practitioner under appropriate supervision in accordance with professional standards of care used with regard to the unique circumstances that apply in each practice situation. Care has been taken to confirm the accuracy of information presented and to describe generally accepted practices. However, the authors, editors, and publisher cannot accept any responsibility for errors or omissions or for any consequences from application of the information in this book and make no warranty, express or implied, with respect to the contents of the book.

Preface

This Instructor's Resource Manual is designed to assist nursing faculty who use the text *Community Health Nursing: Concepts and Practice*, Fifth Edition, by Judith A. Allender, RN,C, MSN, EdD and Barbara W. Spradley, RN, MN. It provides suggestions for enhancing both classroom and clinical laboratory learning of the concepts presented in the accompanying textbook.

The chapters in this resource manual correlate with the chapters in the textbook. Each chapter includes learning objectives, key terms, teaching strategies for the classroom and clinical laboratory settings, ways to use the Activities to Promote Critical Thinking from the textbook in class, and evaluation strategies—multiple-choice questions, essay questions, and individual and group projects.

The *learning objectives* are stated in behavioral terms and reflect the most important concepts presented in the corresponding textbook chapter. These objectives may be used by faculty members in preparing course syllabi or lesson plans or distributed as study guides for students. *Key terms* are identified to assist faculty members in preparing classroom content or terminology worksheets for students.

The *teaching strategies* section includes suggestions for both classroom and clinical laboratory teaching, with a focus on enhancing critical thinking. The *classroom strategies* illustrate and amplify concepts presented in the text. A variety of suggestions are provided to give an educator latitude to choose those that seem most appropriate for her or his own group of students. The strategies include ideas for role playing, simulation gaming, class discussion, and group and individual activities, as well as suggestions for guest speakers and panel discussions by experts in the community. The *clinical laboratory strategies* provide ideas for experiential activities aimed at reinforcing classroom teaching and promoting critical thinking. Again, inclusion of a variety of experiences and settings gives faculty members a wide choice when planning clinical activities.

A feature in the textbook called *Activities to Promote Critical Thinking* is designed to encourage students to enrich their learning of the content in the specific chapter. It is suggested that you provide some of these activities for students within the classroom setting. To enable you to transfer these activities from a solo student activity to the classroom, ways to use them in class, in addition to having them completed by individual students, have been included.

The *evaluation strategies,* which stem from the learning objectives, consist of questions designed to promote critical thinking and evaluate students' understanding of the major concepts in each chapter. Evaluation strategies are presented through multiple-choice and essay questions and individual or group project ideas. They may be used to review content, as part of a formative evaluation, or as part of a summative evaluation in a graded examination. Answers and rationale for the multiple-choice answer choices are provided within each question. The first answer choice listed is the correct one. Each answer choice has rationale why it is correct or incorrect.

It is hoped that faculty members who use this resource manual along with the fifth edition of the textbook will find ideas to help them develop creative teaching strategies and effective evaluation methods, thus enhancing student learning.

I wish to acknowledge the editing and design staff members who have assisted in the preparation of this resource manual, especially Doris Wray, Ancillary Editor, and Margaret Zuccarini, Senior Editor of the accompanying textbook *Community Health Nursing: Concepts and Practice*.

Judith A. Allender

Contents

UNIT I

Foundations of Community Health Nursing

CHAPTER 1

Opportunities and Challenges of Community Health Nursing

LEARNING OBJECTIVES

Upon mastery of this chapter, you should be able to:

■ Define community health and distinguish it from public health.

■ Explain the concept of community.

■ Describe three types of communities.

■ Diagram the health continuum.

■ Differentiate between the three levels of prevention.

■ Analyze six components of community health practice.

■ Describe eight characteristics of community health nursing.

KEY TERMS

Aggregate	Health promotion
Biostatistics	Illness
Collaboration	Population
Common-interest community	Population-focused
Community	Primary prevention
Community health	Public health
Community health nursing	Public health nursing
Community of solution	Rehabilitation
Continuous needs	Research
Epidemiology	Secondary prevention
Episodic needs	Self-care
Evaluation	Self-care deficit
Geographic community	Tertiary prevention
Health	Wellness
Health continuum	

■ Teaching Strategies

CLASSROOM TEACHING STRATEGIES

1. Suggest that the students answer the question, "What is a community?" Put all ideas on the board or on a transparency and discuss. Do all suggestions meet the definition of a community? Why and why not?

2. Use the categories of community discussed in this chapter. Ask the students to categorize as many "communities" as they can. Discuss why they fall into each category.

3. Suggest that the students identify and discuss the opportunities and challenges in the field of community health nursing—before they have experienced many clinical days.

4. Using the following examples, discuss with the students what level of prevention each represents and why:

   a. Teaching infant care to a group of pregnant women

   b. Volunteering to give flu shots at an immunization clinic

   c. Working at a first-aid booth at the local high school football game

   d. Encouraging women to practice monthly breast exams

   e. Working in the shelter after a flood affects many hometown neighbors

   f. Encouraging a post-MI client to continue to take 2-mile walks daily

CLINICAL LABORATORY TEACHING STRATEGIES

1. During a clinical post-conference ask students to identify examples of primary, secondary, and tertiary prevention they were involved in today.

2. Discuss how an experience in the clinical laboratory can be seen as an opportunity or as a challenge. Use examples such as teaching parenting to a new mother, reporting a suspected child abuse case, or interacting with elders at a senior center.

3. Suggest that the students place their clients on the wellness–illness continuum and defend why they placed them where they did.

■ Activities to Promote Critical Thinking in the Classroom

1. Use the clinical laboratory site or the college/university campus as examples. Suggest to the students how the community of nursing students could meet the definition of community.

2. Use clients from the clinical laboratory experience that all students are familiar with or local groups identified/discussed in your daily newspaper. Suggest that the students use two of their own family members and pair up with a peer to discuss why each placed the selected relatives at points on the continuum.

3. Using any of the three groups, families, or individuals chosen in question 2, describe an action for each level of prevention that could be used appropriately to move each closer to optimal wellness.

4. Bring a copy of your local newspaper to class and locate an article written about a community health problem. Use this as the problem of choice and break it down into the three levels of prevention. Identify what role the community health nurse could take in each level of prevention. Repeat this exercise with several problems if the paper contains more than one such story. Ask the students whether they are aware of an ongoing community health problem in their town and use their examples as the topic to be analyzed.

5. Take the steps in question 4 further and discuss a health promotion effort you could use with each population presented.

6. Ask the students to conduct this exercise at home and then bring in their examples during a later class. Share the different topics selected to give the class a broad view of the types of problems, variety of sources available on the Internet for this type of information, and possible solutions community health nursing students can generate.

7. Suggest that the students share in class where they placed themselves on the health continuum and why. Select just three or four to share, based on their willingness. This exercise may reveal information not all students would want to share.

8. Review the eight characteristics of community health nursing described on pages 15 to 19 with the class. Suggest the students give examples of how they have seen community health nurses demonstrate meeting each characteristic. This

exercise is best done 4 to 5 weeks into their clinical laboratory experience when they have had a chance to observe practicing community health nurses.

■ Evaluation Strategies

MULTIPLE-CHOICE QUESTIONS

1. A community of solution is best described as a(n):

   Group of people who solve a problem that affects them
   A community of solution is represented by a group of people with solutions to a problem that affects them all and may come from a variety of geographic communities.

   Community with well-defined geographical boundaries
   This is an example of a geographical community.

   Community with diverse members and interests within a defined area
   This is an example of a geographical community.

   Location served by county and/or state health departments
   This is a regional community or a service community and fits the broad general definition of community.

2. Rehabilitation and long-term follow-up is an example of:

   Tertiary prevention
   Once an insult or injury has occurred, the long-term follow-up and the health care services needed to restore health or maximize functioning are considered tertiary prevention.

   Secondary prevention
   This is identified by early diagnosis and prompt treatment.

   Primary prevention
   This is identified by taking measures to place the body in a state of wellness so that disease and injury do not occur.

   Health promotion
   This term usually refers to the activities taken to promote wellness, prior to any illness or injury.

3. A group of community health nursing students conducted a scoliosis screening program at a junior high school. This type of program is an example of:

   Secondary prevention
   This is identified by early diagnosis and prompt treatment, which is the purpose of a scoliosis screening program.

Tertiary prevention
Once an insult or injury has occurred, the long-term follow-up and the health care services needed to restore health or maximize functioning are considered tertiary prevention.

Corrective action
This is action taken to correct a health care problem and may be part of an additional step if there are students who are found with scoliosis, but it is not part of the screening program.

Primary prevention
This is identified by taking measures to place the body in a state of wellness so that disease and injury do not occur.

4. Community health nursing can best be characterized by the following definition:

It is a field of nursing that combines nursing with public health principles.
This is a brief description of the main characteristics of community health nursing.
Community health nursing focuses on working with individuals in the community.
Community health nursing's focus is on populations, aggregates, and groups.
It is a field of nursing that emphasizes the technical and psychomotor skills of the nurse.
It does not focus on these nursing skills, it focuses on prevention, health promotion, and wellness.
Community health nursing focuses on solo practice and rarely includes working closely with others.
Community health nursing focuses on inter-professional collaboration, which involves working closely with many others.

5. The town of Gaithersburg is a residential part of a national recreational area. It has 3,000 residents and comprises 26 square miles. It has a bank, grocery store, elementary school, gas station, and several small boutiques. It has no clinic or hospital. This could be defined as a:

Geographic community
The data given support the location and parameters of the identified town, thus describing a geographic community.
Community of solution
No data given support that it is a community of solution—one where a group of people come together to solve a problem common to all of them.
Common-interest community
This is a community identified by a common interest or goal. No information is given to indicate this.

Medical trade area
Because it has no medical services identified, it is part of some large medical trade area in order for the people to receive needed medical services. However, Gaithersburg is not a medical trade area itself.

ESSAY QUESTIONS

1. Design a health promotion program for yourself. Identify areas needing improvement in your health; make recommendations, outline goals, and include a time line for accomplishing this program.

2. Place the community you live in on the health continuum. Why did you place it where you did? What areas need to be changed to move it to a higher level of wellness? What can *you* do about it as a community health nursing student?

3. Select clinical examples of a primary, secondary, and tertiary prevention activity that you could engage in during the community health nursing clinical laboratory and discuss your role in the activity.

INDIVIDUAL OR GROUP PROJECTS

1. Attend a city council or county board of supervisors meeting where community leaders are discussing a change that might affect the health of your community. Analyze how the changes may affect the community. If they allow discussion from citizens during the meeting, contribute your thoughts on the effects of the proposed change.

2. Identify a community problem that a group of student nurses in the community health nursing clinical laboratory could solve. As a group, plan to solve the problem working with appropriate community members. Raise the needed funds, establish roles for each student, develop a time line, and complete the project. (As a record of the project, take a series of before and after photographs or photograph the event and give a set of photos to the agency involved in the project.)

CHAPTER 2

Evolution of Community Health Nursing

LEARNING OBJECTIVES

Upon mastery of this chapter, you should be able to:

- Describe the four stages of community health nursing's development.

- Analyze the impact of societal influences on the development and practice of community health nursing.

- Explore the academic and advanced professional preparation of community health nurses.

KEY TERMS

Causal thinking
Community-based nursing
District nursing

■ Teaching Strategies

CLASSROOM TEACHING STRATEGIES

1. Trace the history of community health nursing and discuss the confusion that has arisen about the definitions of community health nursing and public health nursing. Which name do you think best describes this type of nursing?

2. There were only a few early community health nursing leaders discussed in this chapter on the evolution of community health nursing. Go to the Internet or library and research other names that stand out in the history of community health nursing. During a classroom discussion list their contributions. Which general stage of development (early home care nursing, district nursing, public health nursing, or community health nursing) did they contribute to the most?

CLINICAL LABORATORY TEACHING STRATEGIES

1. About halfway through the community health nursing clinical experience, elicit from the students which general stage of development mostly describes the kind of nursing they are doing in the clinical setting. If it is not community health nursing, what changes need to be made to bring the nursing care forward?

2. Ask some of the more experienced community health nurses in the agency you are using for your community health nursing clinical experience (those with 15 or more years of community health experience) how their roles have changed in the past 10 to 20 years. What has changed—agency structure, paperwork expectations, client needs, others? How have the nurses adapted to these changes?

ACTIVITIES TO PROMOTE CRITICAL THINKING IN THE CLASSROOM

1. Select a current major societal influence—such as the limitations of Medicare, the increasing numbers of aging persons, 20% of the country not being covered by health insurance, life-extending drugs that create a population of people living with AIDs (PLWA), and one-fifth of the country's children living in poverty—and discuss how they impact community health nursing differently (or the same) as the societal influences nurses experienced 100 years ago. There are many societal influences. Select some that affect your local community especially hard and are clear to everyone, as well as others that seem to be so far away that they appear to have little influence on local issues. Describe how they really do influence us locally. As an example, civil war in an African country creates additional poverty, stress, illness, and refugees. The refugees cause strain on other nations and brings illness to them. This increases immigration and the potential for diseases to be brought to the new country... and the U.S. may be that country... and your community their new home.

2. Using the historical community health nursing leaders the students found on a solo Internet search, discuss these nurses' approaches or contributions to solving today's population-based issues.

3. Using the sites that the students will use for their clinical laboratory practicum, select a typical client for discussion and identify assessment and intervention methods that would indicate an aggregate or population-focused approach to working with the client. Have the students identify self-care practices they might encourage or teach.

4. Compare and contrast the various population-based programs that are offered by the community health agencies you and the class are aware of or that are provided by the agencies used as clinical laboratory sites. Do you find overlapping services or gaps in services? Share your findings with appropriate community health agency leaders for their feedback.

5. In addition to discussing the advanced nursing options available in your college, university, or neighboring university, what advanced degrees are available in other college departments that might be useful to community health nurses? Suggest students bring brochures of various programs—such as business, health science, or social work—that might be useful additional degrees for a bachelor's-prepared community health nurse. Discuss how and why these degrees could be useful.

■ Evaluation Strategies

MULTIPLE-CHOICE QUESTIONS

1. From 1970 to the present, this era has been known as community health nursing. Which of the following contributed most to this change?

   The settings and the nurses delivering health care in the community
   The numbers, increasing variety of settings, and many nurses coming to work in the community settings since the 1970s have made the most significant difference. Professional associations supported the broader term of community health nursing.

   Decisions made by the American Nurses Association
   Professional agencies supported the change but did not initiate the change–the settings and the nurses delivering the care created the change.

   Decisions made by physicians in a variety of community settings
   Physicians did not contribute to the decision to change the term public health nursing to community health nursing.

   Political conservatism and the desire to eliminate the word "public" from health services
   No political pressure contributed to changing the term public health nursing to community health nursing.

2. The major difference between community health nursing and community-based nursing is:

   Community health nursing focuses on the health of populations, whereas community-based nursing focuses on where the nursing care is delivered.
   This answer describes the major differences when defining these two terms that are often confused.

   Community health nursing focuses on well people, whereas community-based nursing focuses on ill people.
   All people in the community can be placed somewhere along a health continuum whether they are served by community health nurses or community-based nurses.

   Just a matter of preference, as the terms can be used interchangeably.
   The terms mean different things and should not be used interchangeably.

   Community health nursing pertains to nurses working in official agencies, whereas community-based nurses work in for-profit agencies.
   Community health nursing focuses on the health of populations, whereas community-based nursing focuses on where the nursing care is delivered–official, nonprofit, or for-profit.

3. Early home care nursing, before the mid-1800s, was earmarked by:

   Religious orders, friends, and family caring for the sick at home
   These were the three groups providing needed health care to individuals in the community before the mid-1800s.

   Major technical advances with the Industrial Revolution making major changes
   The Industrial Revolution occurred after the 1850s, and technical advances only began to change health care in the 1900s.

   The accomplishments stemming from the work of Florence Nightingale
   Florence Nightingale was born in 1820 and was first known for her work during the Crimean War (1854–1856). She was not a major influence on early home care nursing before 1850.

Conquering infectious diseases, public health, and maternal-child health programs
These types of changes occurred in the late 1800s and first half of the 1900s; they did not occur before the mid-1800s.

4. There have been six recent (last 30–40 years) major societal influences on the growth of community health nursing, discussed in Chapter 2. Three significant ones are:

Progress in causal thinking, changes in education, and the role of women
These are three of the six major influences. The other three are technical advances, the consumer movement, and economic forces.

Increase in the world population, progress in communicable disease control, and advances in industrial development
World population has been increasing for the last century, doubling every 30 years; we made our greatest strides in communicable disease control in the first 70 years of the 20th century; and we advanced in industrial development from 1850 to 1950.

Increase in the birth rate, advances in world exploration, and emerging political forces
The birth rate has been decreasing per woman of childbearing age in the past 30 years; the world was explored primarily in the 1400s to 1600s; and there are always emerging political forces, none recently having more significance than others.

Self-care movement, recognition of the germ theory, and the Industrial Revolution
The self-care movement is progressing slowly and has not significantly changed the role of community health nurses. The germ theory and Industrial Revolution occurred from 1850 to 1900.

5. The contributions of Lillian Wald to the advancement of community health nursing were enormous. Some of the accomplishments she is known for include:

Establishing family-centered nursing and outreach services in New York City at the turn of the 20th century
Lillian Wald worked with immigrant families in the Lower East Side of New York City, providing home visits, a neighborhood center, and general sanitation improvement for families and health care services to children in schools.

Bringing clean and safe nursing practice to soldiers during the Crimean War in the 1850s
This describes some of the work of Florence Nightingale.

Helping high-risk populations who were experiencing tropical diseases in Central America and the Caribbean in the late 1800s
This describes some of the work of Mary Seacole.

Establishing home nursing services in London, beginning District Nursing Services in the 1860s
This describes some of the work of William Rathbone, Florence Nightingale, and Florence Lees.

ESSAY QUESTIONS

1. You are a nursing colleague of Lillian Wald, early in the 20th century. Describe what nursing in the immigrant neighborhoods of New York City is like. Describe how it feels to be a nurse at that time.

2. Describe how advances in technology have affected community health nursing in the past 20 years. How do you picture technology affecting community health nursing in the future?

INDIVIDUAL OR GROUP PROJECTS

1. Have four groups of students design community health nursing care for the same hypothetical family. Each group imagines they are working at a different time in history and designs care accordingly.
   a. Early home care nursing stage—before mid-1800s
   b. The district nursing stage—mid-1800s to 1900
   c. The public health nursing stage—1900 to 1970
   d. The community health nursing stage—1970 to present

2. Offer the opportunity for students to select a community health nurse from history and research her or his life and works. Students may select the nurse based on race, culture, location, works, or time in history. Allow class time for sharing brief summaries of the nurses' works and times.

CHAPTER 3

Roles and Settings for Community Health Nursing Practice

LEARNING OBJECTIVES

Upon mastery of this chapter, you should be able to:

- Identify the three core public health functions basic to community health nursing.

- Describe and differentiate among seven different roles of the community health nurse.

- Discuss the seven roles within the framework of public health nursing functions.

- Explain the importance of each role for influencing people's health.

- Identify and discuss factors that affect a nurse's selection and practice of each role.

- Describe seven settings in which community health nurses practice.

- Discuss the nature of community health nursing and the common threads basic to its practice, woven throughout all roles and settings.

- Identify principles of sound nursing practice in the community.

KEY TERMS

Advocate	Human skills
Assessment	Leader
Assurance	Managed care
Case management	Manager
Clinician	Organizer
Collaborator	Planner
Conceptual skills	Policy development
Controller	Researcher
Educator	Technical skills
Evaluator	

■ Teaching Strategies

CLASSROOM TEACHING STRATEGIES

1. Invite a panel of community health nurses who practice in a variety of settings and assume various roles to speak to the class. Ask the nurses to discuss each of the seven major roles according to the importance that is placed on each in their particular setting. Allow time for questions from the students after the presentation.

2. Find some copies of old nursing journals (1925–1945) and share the role expectations of nurses working in the community 50 or more years ago with today's roles. Suggest the students do this activity in class or prepare your lesson plans from the old journals and lead the discussion yourself. Do you notice a difference in roles during the WWII years 1941 to 1945?

CLINICAL LABORATORY TEACHING STRATEGIES

1. At their assigned clinical practice site, have the community health nursing students examine the major roles needed by nurses practicing at that or similar settings.

2. During a clinical conference, near the end of the clinical laboratory experience, ask the community health nursing students to share examples of how they carried out the major roles of community health nursing, using examples from the work they did during the course.

ACTIVITIES TO PROMOTE CRITICAL THINKING IN THE CLASSROOM

1. Identify the populations the students will be working with in their clinical laboratory experience this term. Discuss how the students can make nursing services holistic and focused on wellness.

2. Select several community health nursing roles and have students identify how they could apply the roles while meeting the needs of familiar people they all know: a movie star, a sports figure, a local politician, or you (if you are brave).

3. Create some hypothetical situations and have the students describe how a community health nurse would combine a variety of roles described on pages 41 to 49. Examples might include a community health nurse working with:

   a. A South American Indian tribe in remote Argentina

   b. Women released from prison

   c. An inner city neighborhood with obvious gang activity

4. Have the students discuss the similarities and differences between or among the various clinical laboratory sites they are using this term. Are the community health nursing roles used the same or very different? Why or why not?

5. Ask the students what roles they have been using with the populations they are serving in community health nursing clinical laboratory this term. How could they expand these roles to be more aggregate focused? Suggest that they try to stretch their practice approaches to be more aggregate focused. Give them suggestions on how this can be accomplished, knowing the sites used, populations served, agency philosophies, and student abilities.

6. Have the students bring the consumer-focused health-related information they found on the Internet or in the library to class. Place all of it on a table in the room so the students can peruse the information and see the sources and quality of information. Encourage them to use the information to enhance their own client resources.

7. Locate a piece of research that was done collaboratively—among faculty in the nursing department or across disciplines with faculty from other departments, colleges, or schools. The Research and Grants office on campus would be a good resource if there is no current research you are aware of. Make copies of the research abstract for students to use in discussion. Answer the questions found in this question in the textbook on page 54. Better yet, describe your research with colleagues from nursing or with other professionals from campus or the larger community and have the students respond to it using the same questions on page 54 for question 7.

■ Evaluation Strategies

MULTIPLE-CHOICE QUESTIONS

1. Jonathan DeLow, a community health nurse, collected data for several months on the birth weights of newborns to mothers who smoked throughout their pregnancy. This is an example of which of the following roles?

   Researcher
   Collecting data is one of the steps in the research process. This is the role most clearly identified in the example.

   Collaborator
   This is defined by working with a variety of colleagues to benefit client care. This role is not demonstrated in the example.

   Manager
   When functioning in the manager role, the nurse exercises administrative direction toward the accomplishment of specified goals. This role is not demonstrated in the example.

   Clinician
   The nurse ensures that health services are provided not just to individuals and families but also to groups and populations. This role is not demonstrated in the example.

2. Mr. DeLow spends much of his time as a community health nurse working with police officers, social workers, health educators, and other nurses. This is an example of his role as a:

   Collaborator
   This is defined by working with a variety of colleagues to benefit client care. This is the role most clearly identified in the example.

   Clinician
   The nurse ensures that health services are provided not just to individuals and families but also to groups and populations. This role is not demonstrated in the example.

   Educator
   The nurse acts as a health educator to individuals, families, groups, aggregates, and populations. This role is not demonstrated in the example.

   Researcher
   Collecting data is one of the steps in the research process. This role is not demonstrated in the example.

3. Mr. DeLow makes home visits to families, holds immunization clinics for infants and children, and sets up flu-shot clinics for elders. This is an example of the role of:

Clinician
These are examples of the role of clinician: observing, listening, counseling, and providing a physical nursing service.

Educator
The nurse acts as a health educator to individuals, families, groups, aggregates, and populations. This role is not demonstrated in the example.

Advocate
As an advocate, the nurse speaks for clients or acts on their behalf to get needed action and services. This role is not demonstrated in the example.

Manager
When functioning in the manager role, the nurse exercises administrative direction toward the accomplishment of specified goals. This role is not demonstrated in the example.

4. When Mr. DeLow organizes his day, plans client care, leads staff conferences, and supervises a new staff member, he is fulfilling the role of:

Manager
When functioning in the manager role, the nurse exercises administrative direction toward the accomplishment of specified goals. This is the role most clearly identified in the example.

Advocate
As an advoce, the nurse speaks for clients or acts on their behalf to get needed action and services. This role is not demonstrated in the example.

Collaborator
This is defined by working with a variety of colleagues to benefit client care. This role is not demonstrated in the example.

Researcher
Collecting data is one of the steps in the research process. This role is not demonstrated in the example.

5. Sara Dukell, a community health nurse, works with a religious community, assessing, diagnosing, implementing, and evaluating care that the community members need. This setting provides her the opportunity to be involved with:

Parish nursing
The example describes parish nursing—providing nursing services to a religious community based on their beliefs, traditions, and tenets.

Occupational health nursing
Occupational health nurses provide health promotion, health education, first aid, and restorative services to employees in business and industry. This role is not demonstrated in the example.

School nursing
School nurses provide health promotion, health education, and first aid to students in schools and colleges. This role is not demonstrated in the example.

Residential institution nursing
Community health nurses who practice residential institution nursing provide health promotion, health education, and health maintenance services to groups of people living in institutions, such as the elderly, disabled, and incarcerated. This role is not demonstrated in the example.

6. There are three primary functions of public health: assessment, policy development, and assurance. Community health nursing incorporates each one as they are fundamental to all roles within the realm of practice. The following is an example of assurance:

The community health nurse is involved in the activities that make certain that services are provided.
This is the description of assurance.

The community health nurse gathers and analyzes information that will affect the health of the people to be served.
This is a description of assessment.

The community health nurse provides leadership in convening and facilitating community groups toward meeting their needs, often involving changes in and additions to existing laws.
This is a definition of policy development.

The community health nurse accesses relevant data that enable him or her to identify strengths, weaknesses, and needs within the community.
This is a description of assessment.

ESSAY QUESTIONS

1. Select one of the seven major roles of the community health nurse and develop it fully, using client foci and services offered. Use the clinical laboratory setting in which you have community health nursing as an example.

2. Select one of the seven settings in which community health nurses practice and develop the nurse's role of *educator* in that setting.

INDIVIDUAL OR GROUP PROJECTS

1. Have the students select a practice setting of their choice (be sure all settings are selected at least once) and suggest that they observe a nurse in the chosen setting. The student should be prepared to discuss the nurse's role during a class later in the term. This activity can be formalized by you making the contacts, having clinical time set aside for the activity, setting up possible observation sites yourself, and expecting a worksheet completed by the student after the experience and signed by the nurse observed. Alternatively, it can be set up by the students on their own time with no formal paperwork, just a journal entry.

2. Have the students identify the major employers in the community where the nursing program is located. Select the top 10 employers who do not have an occupational health nurse. Have small (two to three) groups of students meet with the safety director, public relations representative, or manager. Ask the company representative what they think a nurse could do for their company if they employed one. If the response is limited, the students should educate the representative on what a nurse could do for the company. Use the seven major roles to build examples. Report the variety of responses to the entire class.

CHAPTER 4

Transcultural Nursing in the Community

LEARNING OBJECTIVES

Upon mastery of this chapter, you should be able to:

- Define and explain the concept of culture.

- Discuss the meaning of cultural diversity and its significance for community health nursing.

- Describe the meaning and effects of ethnocentrism on community health nursing practice.

- Identify five characteristics shared by all cultures.

- Contrast the health-related values, beliefs, and practices of culturally diverse populations with those of the dominant U.S. culture.

- Conduct a cultural assessment.

- Apply transcultural nursing principles in community health nursing practice.

KEY TERMS

Cultural assessment	Ethnicity
Cultural diversity	Ethnocentrism
Cultural relativism	Microculture
Cultural self-awareness	Minority group
Cultural sensitivity	Race
Culture	Subcultures
Culture shock	Tacit
Dominant values	Transcultural nursing
Enculturation	Value
Ethnic group	

■Teaching Strategies

CLASSROOM TEACHING STRATEGIES

1. Ask a representative from one of the cultural groups in your local community (or one of the students in the community health nursing class) to speak to the class about various aspects of his or her culture. The Cultural Assessment Guide (Table 4-5) could be used by the speaker.

2. Invite a panel made up of representatives of the cultural groups in your community to class to speak. This group may also be helped by the Cultural Assessment Guide (Table 4-5), either in its original form or a modified one.

CLINICAL LABORATORY TEACHING STRATEGIES

1. Have students present a cultural assessment of their own family. To highlight their presentations, suggest they bring photographs of their family members, interesting family documents (citizenship papers, Daughters of the American Revolution documents, etc.), or other meaningful family memorabilia.

2. Have students complete a cultural assessment on one of their assigned families that represent a specific cultural community or one that helps to broaden the definition of diversity (a minority ethnic group, a family living in poverty, the disabled). Share with peers in a community health nursing clinical laboratory conference, perhaps as part of a case study.

ACTIVITIES TO PROMOTE CRITICAL THINKING IN THE CLASSROOM

1. Suggest the students share some of their own cultural experiences when confronted with a different culture, while they were vacationing or visiting in another country, as a new resident in a different region of the country, or as a new immigrant to the U.S. What aspects of their day-to-day living were impacted by the cultural differences? How did it feel to be a minority among the local majority? What parenting, health, dietary or other practices did they notice that were different from their own?

2. Have the class of students share tacit (pages 61—62) cultural rules from their own family. Are there more differences or similarities? Discuss these differences and similarities. Were they expected or did the students think they would be more alike or more different?

3. Select a variety of groups to share with the students that they may have collectively encountered at some time in their life, such as a group of homeless men, Native Americans at a pow-wow, a group of Chinese acrobats, Buddhist monks, or a group of Catholic nuns. Suggest the students use Bennet's stages of cross-cultural sensitivity on page 60 to determine their own feelings about groups of people the class has knowledge of in common.

4. Select a population group that all students will be working with this term. This might be an ethnic group, an age group, or a social-economic group, such as Asian Americans, elders, or people living in poverty. What appropriate information will students need to gather to provide culturally relevant nursing services? What sources will they tap?

5. Have the students share cultural practices from community groups they care for in their clinical laboratory experiences. Discuss these practices. Determine whether they are healthy, safe, neutral, harmful, life-threatening, etc. If the practices seem unsafe or unhealthy, discuss with the students interventions that will help modify behaviors without disrupting cultural norms.

6. Suggest that the students complete this activity and make copies of their findings. Keep these resources in a large file in your office, student lounge, or other accessible place where all students will have them available for their own reference.

7. Suggest that the students complete this activity in small groups so that there are 7 to 10 different disciplines represented. Use class time to have student groups share the contributions of this professional in the caregiving of aggregates in the community.

■ Evaluation Strategies

MULTIPLE-CHOICE QUESTIONS

1. You overhear a neighbor say, "I don't understand why the Yang's take their young teenage daughters to the Hmong New Year celebration and have them play these match-making games. The girls are too young to be looking for husbands." Which of the following would be the most appropriate response?

"Every culture has its differences; I think it is valuable that the Yang's are keeping their cultural practices alive."
This response recognizes and values cultural differences.

"The Yang's are very different from us; maybe in time we can convince them that their practices are not right."
This response comes from an ethnocentric viewpoint and is not the most appropriate.

"I know what you mean, I was thinking the same thing. You wouldn't catch me doing something similar with my teens."
This response demonstrates and reinforces strong ethnocentric views and is not the most appropriate.

"I feel sorry for the Yang's girls, they must feel funny in those cultural costumes. Perhaps we should talk to the parents and convince them how teens in America feel about such things."
This response sounds as though it is intended to be helpful, but it also reinforces an ethnocentric viewpoint and is not the most appropriate response.

2. When we say that "culture is tacit," this means:

Culture is mostly unexpressed and is at the unconscious level.
This is the definition of the term tacit, which is used to help explain how culture provides an implicit set of cues for behavior and is one of the characteristics of culture.

Patterns of cultural behavior are acquired and are not inherited.
This explains how cultural practices are learned, another characteristic of culture.

Culture is a functional and integrated whole.
This states that cultural practices are integrated and are not just an assortment of various customs and traits.

Cultures undergo changes and do not remain static.
This demonstrates that culture is dynamic, another characteristic of culture.

3. The complexion of the United States is changing. Over 30% of immigrants coming to the U.S., especially in the last 5 to 10 years, come from:

Mexico and the Caribbean
In 1996, 18% and 13% (31%) came from Mexico and the Caribbean, respectively.

Asia
From all of the Asian countries, immigration amounted to 27% of newcomers in 1998.

Europe
From all of the European countries, immigration amounted to 17% of newcomers in 1998.

Africa
From all of the African countries, immigration amounted to 5% of newcomers in 1996.

4. Native American cultural similarities include:

Respect for advancing age and elders
This is a common cultural similarity among Native Americans.

Concern for the distant future
Native Americans as a group live in the present and do not focus on the distant future.

Encouragement and value of competition
Native Americans are more apt to value generosity and sharing and discourage competition.

Value of the spoken word through frequent dialogue and discussion
Native Americans practice periods of silence and value thoughtful speech.

5. In the Interaction Model of viewing people with disabilities, a person with a disability is seen as:

Different
This views a disability as being neutral, that is, being different is neither right nor wrong, good nor bad—just different.

Deficient
This view comes from the medical model in which a disability is a deficiency or an abnormality.

Abnormal
This view comes from the medical model in which a disability is a deficiency or an abnormality.

Negative
This view comes from the medical model in which a disability is a deficiency or an abnormality and thus is negative.

6. Nurses should follow transcultural nursing principles. One of the first is to develop cultural self-awareness by:

Examining one's own culture carefully and becoming aware that alternative viewpoints are possible
This is essential to becoming culturally aware and engaging successfully in transcultural nursing.

Recognizing that culturally based values, beliefs, and practices influence people's health and life styles
This is the second step in developing transcultural nursing principles—cultivating cultural sensitivity.

Obtaining health-related information about a designated cultural group concerning their values, beliefs, and practices
This is the third step in developing transcultural nursing principles–assessing a client group's culture.

Showing respect and patience while learning about other cultures
This is the fourth step in developing transcultural nursing principles–key behaviors for the nurse to practice during the cultural learning process.

ESSAY QUESTIONS

1. Select one of the following cultural values: food, religion, parenting, or health practices. Compare and contrast your behavior/beliefs in the selected area with someone from a cultural group different than yours.

2. Select one category of the Cultural Assessment Guide (Table 4-5) and develop a response using the sample data ideas. Describe these data in relation to your family of origin and how you (as an adult) view the same category.

INDIVIDUAL OR GROUP PROJECTS

1. Plan a poster session in which each of the students designs a poster depicting aspects of one culture in the local community (assign groups of students to do this if there are not enough cultures and subcultures to assign one to each student).

2. Plan a film festival. Have the students locate several good films depicting different cultures. Have a tasting party of ethnic food eaten by these groups.

3. Have each student share a short and interesting story about their own culture. Often in a group of students, if there are distinctly different cultural groups represented, students from Northern European backgrounds with families who have lived in the U.S. for generations may feel that they "have no culture" because their skin is the same color and they dress alike. Reinforce each student's family uniqueness by having them share the subtleties of their own family's cultural practices. This might take the form of an old family food recipe, how religious holidays are celebrated, or how family members view the work ethic or interact with elders or children in the family.

CHAPTER 5

Values and Ethics in Community Health Nursing

LEARNING OBJECTIVES

Upon mastery of this chapter, you should be able to:

- Describe the nature of values and value systems and their influence on community health.

- Identify personal and professional values that you bring to decision-making with and for community health clients.

- Articulate the impact of key values on professional decision-making.

- Discuss the application of ethical principles to community health nursing decision-making.

- Use a decision-making process with and for community health clients that incorporates values and ethical principles.

KEY TERMS

Autonomy	Moral evaluations
Beneficence	Nonmaleficence
Distributive justice	Respect
Egalitarian justice	Restorative justice
Equity	Self-determination
Ethical decision-making	Self-interest
Ethical dilemma	Terminal values
Ethics	Value
Fidelity	Value systems
Instrumental values	Values clarification
Justice	Veracity
Moral	Well-being

■ Teaching Strategies

CLASSROOM TEACHING STRATEGIES

1. Assign the students to complete the first activity in the Activities to Promote Critical Thinking at the end of Chapter 5 prior to the lecture/discussion of this chapter. Ask for volunteers to share their responses. (Note: Be prepared to give examples of typical responses if the student choose to share in a very limited fashion.)

2. Provide the students with a brief case study that involves making an ethical decision. Find examples from the national, regional, or local media. Some situations have been in the media for months and serve as extreme examples.

CLINICAL LABORATORY TEACHING STRATEGIES

1. Have the students identify actual or potential situations that could require the need for ethical decision making. Ask students to briefly describe one situation in their clinical journal (log or diary) or share one verbally in clinical post-conference.

2. Ask students to discuss with a trusted peer or community health nurse how the key values of self-determination, well-being, and equity guide her or his decision-making in practitioner–client relationships.

ACTIVITIES TO PROMOTE CRITICAL THINKING IN THE CLASSROOM

1. This activity includes 11 different emotional issues for discussion. Have the class use these issues for a general class discussion or select others of your choice from your particular community, aggregate issues your students deal with in clinical laboratory experiences, or a major international or national issue currently in the news. See whether the class can come to a consensus on feelings about the issues.

2. Have each student select an area of confusion or conflict in community health nursing practice, using the examples from the textbook exercise or selecting ones currently affecting your students' practice. Use a grid similar to the one on page 91 and have the students decide whether their belief reflects one or more of the seven steps in the valuing process (page 83).

3. Place the 11 nursing actions plus a blank space in this activity on the board or an overhead transparency and ask the students to rank them from 1 to 12. Have the students share their responses with the class. Are there similarities? Are there major differences? Discuss what makes them so much alike or different.

4. Suggest the students do this activity in their different clinical laboratory sites and share their experiences with the class. Have the students answer these questions:

   a. Were there values in common?

   b. What ethical principles were used?

   c. What decision-making framework is used by the agency committee?

   d. What would you have liked to contribute to the committee's discussion?

5. Suggest all students complete this activity and bring their findings to class for discussion. Discuss what a community health nurse or student community health nurse could do regarding this impending legislation.

■ Evaluation Strategies

MULTIPLE-CHOICE QUESTIONS

1. Prescriptive-proscriptive beliefs:

   Determine whether an action is desirable
   Prescriptive-proscriptive beliefs determine whether an action is desirable or undesirable. Moral evaluations are prescriptive-prospective beliefs.

   Are non-mental evaluations
   Quite the contrary—prescriptive-proscriptive beliefs are moral evaluations.

   Refer to modes of conduct
   Prescriptive-proscriptive beliefs determine whether an action is desirable or undesirable, which may lead to a mode of conduct, but they are not the modes of conduct themselves.

   Are organized into a hierarchical system
   There is no hierarchy in prescriptive-proscriptive beliefs—they are desirable or undesirable without a leveling of beliefs.

2. One of the basic human values that guides decision making is equity. This value is defined as:

   The belief that like cases should be treated alike and/or treated fairly
   Equity is defined as the value directing like cases to be treated alike and that all individuals be treated fairly.

   The capacity to form, revise, and pursue personal life plans
   This defines the value of self-determination.

   Interventions to promote clients' health and a sense of well-being
   The pursuit of well-being is a value, and when health care practitioners work with clients their intervention activities must be in synchrony with the clients' values.

   The preference for joint decision making over individual decision making
   This is considered a personality trait or a situational preference and is not a value in and of itself.

3. The outcome that can be expected from the basic human value of self-determination is:

   Individual autonomy
   Self-determination promotes individual autonomy and enhances self-concept, health- promoting behaviors, and quality of care.

   A lowered self-concept
   This is not an expected outcome; in fact, the individual autonomy self-determination gives is self-concept building, not lowering.

   Detrimental health behaviors
   This is not an expected outcome of self-determination; however, if someone pursues personal life plans to excess, this could cause ill health.

   A lack of quality care
   This response has nothing to do with self-determination as a value.

4. A bill in the legislature would eliminate a state law that currently funds child health promotion services for low-income children. As a community health nurse you want to work at a primary level of prevention, so you:

   Advocate through active lobbying against the bill and gather community support
   This demonstrates the primary level of prevention by helping to stop the bill from going through the legislature and possibly passing.

   Advocate for amendment to the passed law to allow some funding for children to remain
   This demonstrates secondary prevention—the law has passed and now you are working to amend it.

   Once the bill has passed, seek private resources to support funding of health promotion services for low-income children
   This demonstrates tertiary prevention—the law has passed and you are seeking ways to continue to offer the services that were eliminated.

Gather a group of health professionals to volunteer in the community and provide the health promotion services eliminated by the passed bill *This demonstrates tertiary prevention—the law has passed and you are seeking ways to continue to offer the services that were eliminated.*

ESSAY QUESTIONS

1. Provide the students with a short case study that involves an ethical dilemma and ask them to react to it in writing. Ask that the responses be anonymous. Read the responses and ask for class reactions to the various views shared. (This is a good exercise to stimulate thought, discussion, and participation, not to be graded.)

2. Ask students to share an ethical dilemma they were part of or witnessed in their personal or work life before entering the nursing program. How did they respond to it? How would they respond to it if it were to occur today? Is their response different now? Why?

INDIVIDUAL OR GROUP PROJECTS

1. Have the students participate in a debate. Follow a pre-determined debate format that you select. Allow the students to choose topics appropriate to community health nursing that are currently controversial within the profession or in your local community. Have peers grade each group or contribute to 50% of the overall grade. Rationale for the grade would be given based on criteria you establish.

   Helpful hint: Debate format for one debate in a 50-minute class period

   Have the group work in two teams—pro and con

   Allow 10 minutes for presentation of each side (20 minutes)

   Allow 10 minutes of open questions from the rest of the students (10 minutes)

   Allow 2 minutes from each side to summarize their views (4 minutes)

2. Select item number 3 from the Activities to Promote Critical Thinking for this chapter. Have students rank the 12 items individually, allowing 5 to 6 minutes for the exercise. Then suggest that students work in small groups (select the groups by birthday months, count off by 5s, or use some system so clusters of friends will be in different groups) for 15 minutes to come up with a common ranking reached by consensus. Discuss the difficulty of the individual task versus the group task. What items entailed the greatest concession for students? Why? Why did they concede so much?

CHAPTER 6

Structure and Function of Community Health Services

LEARNING OBJECTIVES

Upon mastery of this chapter, you should be able to:

- Trace historic events and philosophy leading to today's health services delivery.

- Outline the current organizational structure of the public health care system.

- Examine the three core functions of public health as they apply to health services delivery.

- Differentiate between the functions of public versus private sector health care agencies.

- Explain the influence of selected legislative acts in the United States on shaping current health services policy and practice.

- Examine the public health services provided by selected international health organizations.

- Explore how the structure and functions of community health services affect community health nursing practice.

KEY TERMS

Assurance
Core public health
  functions
Department of Health
  and Human Services
Hebrew hygienic code
Medically indigent
Official health agencies
Pan American Health
  Organization Children's
  Emergency Fund

Policy development
Proprietary health
  services
Public Health Service
Quarantine
Sanitation
Shattuck Report
United Nations
  International
Voluntary health agencies
World Health Organization

■ Teaching Strategies

CLASSROOM TEACHING STRATEGIES

1. Lecturing on the important health service acts may not be effective. A better approach may be to have students research selected acts and report on them briefly, including an example of how the act has affected an individual, family, or group the student is aware of.

2. Has a local agency lost funding or received additional funding in your community? If so, discuss how this change will affect health locally or regionally.

3. Invite a speaker from the local Social Security office to speak to the class about services provided and the requirements that must be met for such services.

CLINICAL LABORATORY TEACHING STRATEGIES

1. Suggest that each student secure an organizational chart from a local health care agency—perhaps from the agency where they have their community health nursing clinical laboratory experience or another agency they interact with. The students should identify the type of agency and compare and contrast the effectiveness of the different structures.

2. Suggest that each student visit a health service agency in the community and describe the function of that agency, the population served, and its type (official agency, private practice, private proprietary agency, or voluntary agency). Compile a directory of these agencies for student reference.

3. If your students work in a health care agency during community health clinical laboratory, ask the supervising nurse to share the structure of the agency and how it "fits" into the local health care delivery system. Ask the supervisor to share the benefits and restrictions of such a structure.

ACTIVITIES TO PROMOTE CRITICAL THINKING IN THE CLASSROOM

1. Using the core public health functions of assessment, policy development, and assurance, have the students share what the community health agency, used for clinical laboratory practice, offers its clients compared with those listed on textbook page 100 for local public health agencies. How does the community health nurse incorporate these into her or his role?

2. Have an official from the state health department speak to the class and discuss the services of the department. How do the services described compare with the list on textbook pages 100–101?

3. If you have students working in private health agencies, have them compare the complementary and supplementary functions of these agencies with those listed on textbook page 104. Have the students answer the following: Does the agency work collaboratively with local public agencies? How does the role of the nurse compare with that of nurses in public agencies?

4. Have the students share their Internet findings on international health care issues. Have them discuss these questions: What are some of the current concerns? What are the new or emerging diseases? How can a local community health nurse use such information?

5. Conduct this debate in class using a debate format of your choosing or use a format similar to the following: Divide the class into thirds—pro, con, and observers. Give each side 10 minutes to state its case, followed by 5 minutes of rebuttal. Incorporate time for the observers to ask questions, and conclude with a 2-minute period to have each side summarize its viewpoint.

6. Suggest the students participate in this activity individually and share their findings verbally in class with their peers. Have the students answer the following questions: Are the answers very different among the older adults or the young adults? Are the answers between the groups very different? What are the main themes of concern among those interviewed? Are these issues being addressed in our government or through our local official or private agencies?

■ Evaluation Strategies

MULTIPLE-CHOICE QUESTIONS

1. Official health care agencies are

   Tax supported
   This type of agency is tax supported; thus, it must provide services determined by the federal government or the state.

   Voluntary
   This type of agency is supported by donations or private funds, and no federal, state, or local tax money supports it. Because no tax money supports voluntary agencies, they can provide any services they deem important and needed.

   Proprietary
   A proprietary agency is an extension of another agency and is governed by the policies of the sponsoring agency. An example may be a hospital that has its own home health services.

   Privately supported
   This type of agency is supported by donations or private funds, and no federal, state, or local tax money supports it. Because no tax money supports privately supported agencies, they can provide any services they deem important and needed.

2. The level of health care agency where people actually receive their services is the:

   Local
   Regardless of the level of agency financing the service, it is provided at the local level.

   State
   The state provides few direct services to clients—it does publish pamphlets, but they are distributed at the local level. The state level supports services provided at the local level and filters information and data down from the national and international levels.

   National
   The federal level provides no direct services to clients—it does publish pamphlets, but they are distributed at the local level. The federal/national level financially supports health services provided at the state and local levels and filters information and data down from the international level.

   International
   The international level provides no direct services to clients—it does work with a variety of nations and publish documents of important world health data that clients may order. However, the

international level financially supports health services provided to a country at its local level if that nation cannot deal with the enormity of its health problems.

3. An example of a voluntary organization is the:

American Heart Association
This is a voluntary organization. It gets no federal funds and is privately supported, which makes it a voluntary organization.

The U.S. Public Health Service
This is an official organization. It gets federal funds, which makes it an official organization.

The National Institutes of Health
This is an official organization. It gets federal funds, which makes it an official organization.

Women, Infant, and Children Program (WIC)
This is an official organization. It gets federal funds, which makes it an official organization.

4. The Shattuck Report is considered a landmark document because it made a tremendous impact on:

Sanitary progress and the use of vital statistics in Massachusetts in 1850
This is essentially what the document proposed, when, and where. It was rich with health, disease control, and environmental health strategies.

The speed with which health-focused bills pass the legislature
The Shattuck Report had no affect on the speed of bills passing the legislature.

The organizational structure of the U.S. Public Health Service
The Shattuck Report had no affect on the U.S. Public Health Service's structure.

The Hebrew Hygienic Code
The Shattuck Report was written 2000 years after the Hebrew Hygenic Code and had no affect on it.

5. A major act that passed in 1935 was designed to provide revolutionary welfare insurance and assistance, particularly benefiting high-risk mothers and children. It is called the:

Social Security Act
The Social Security Act was passed in 1935 and began a foundation for supportive services that eventually assists most people in the United States through its various amendments since 1935.

Hill-Burton Act
This act, passed in 1946, was an important breakthrough in nationwide health facilities planning, not social welfare.

Occupational Health and Safety Act
This 1970 act provides protection to workers against personal injury or illness resulting from hazardous working conditions.

Omnibus Budget Reconciliation Act
This 1981 act had a profound effect on public health by substantially reducing funding authorization and the budget and shifting more power to the states.

ESSAY QUESTIONS

1. Select a legislative act passed in the 1900s and discuss how the changes brought about by the act have affected you personally and professionally.

2. Describe what life might have been like 5000 years ago before the need for health care practices was recognized.

3. What health-related bills do you think need to be passed in the next decade? How would passing them affect you personally and professionally? What might you do to initiate the formulation of such a bill?

INDIVIDUAL OR GROUP PROJECTS

1. Suggest groups of students select a legislative act, research its development in depth, analyze it, and share opinions about it with classroom peers.

2. Suggest students write, e-mail, or visit their congressperson or senator, share their opinion on a piece of legislation before the legislature at this time, and ask for the representative's support—pro or con.

CHAPTER 7

Economics of Health Care

LEARNING OBJECTIVES

Upon mastery of this chapter, you should be able to:

- Define the concept of health care economics.

- Describe three sources of health care financing.

- Compare and contrast retrospective and prospective health care payment systems.

- Analyze the issues and trends influencing health care economics and community health services delivery.

- Explain the causes and effects of health care rationing.

- List the pros and cons of managed competition as opposed to a single-payer system.

- Explain the philosophical implications of health care financing patterns on community health nursing's mission and values.

KEY TERMS

Capitation rates	Medicare
Competition	Microeconomic theory
Cost sharing	National health insurance
Diagnosis-related groups	Preferred provider
Gross national product	organization
Health care economics	Prospective payment
Health maintenance	Rationing
organization	Regulation
Macroeconomic theory	Retrospective payment
Managed care	Single-payer system
Managed competition	Third-party payments
Medicaid	Universal coverage

■ Teaching Strategies

Classroom Teaching Strategies

1. Arrange a debate on a current health care issue, such as Medicare cutbacks, medication coverage for elders, or any issue that affects clients locally, regionally, or nationally. Divide the class into debate teams, and set up a debate format that fits in with the time frame. Allow some students to be the "audience." Their responsibility will be to ask both sides pertinent questions at times during the debate format or at the end.

2. Invite the director of nursing from a home health agency to discuss how health care economics affects the functioning of a home health agency.

CLINICAL LABORATORY TEACHING STRATEGIES

1. Invite the director of nursing from the agency where the students have their community health nursing clinical laboratory to talk on health economics and how it affects public health services provided by the agency.

2. Ask the students to assess their clients' health care insurance coverage. What type of system is it (public, private, HMP, PPO)? How do the clients feel about it? Doe it meet their needs? What would they change if they could?

3. Suggest that the students assess their own health care insurance coverage. They should ask themselves the same questions they asked their clients in question 2.

ACTIVITIES TO PROMOTE CRITICAL THINKING IN THE CLASSROOM

1. Have an open discussion regarding public health goals and the goal of health care economics. Ask the students the following: Are the two compatible? Do public health services consider the economics of their services? Could public health services be provided in more cost-effective ways? What are some suggestions for cost savings you have?

2. Ask the students to share their experiences in the clinical laboratory regarding the impact that managed care has had on services provided by the agency. This can be done from the collection of interviews conducted in this activity individually.

3. This activity should first be done alone as a mental exercise. Suggest that the students bring their thoughts on this subject to class and share their views of prospective versus retrospective payment systems. Ask the students whether one method promotes wellness and preventive health care practices more than another.

4. Facilitate this debate in class using a debate format of your choosing or use a format similar to the following: Divide the class into thirds—pro, con, and observers. Give each side 10 minutes to state its case, followed by 5 minutes of rebuttal. Incorporate time for the observers to ask questions, and conclude with a 2-minute period to have each side summarize its viewpoint.

5. Managed care has been the most influential form of health care reform. Has it made improvements (better access, lower cost, higher quality) in our health care delivery system? Use data from articles located by the students to support viewpoints on managed care, health care reform, and public health response.

6. Using the up-to-date information on position statements or legislation affecting public health found by the students, facilitate a discussion on the concerns that these address. Discuss what community health nurses or student community health nurses can do about the issues.

■ Evaluation Strategies

MULTIPLE-CHOICE QUESTIONS

1. The following is true about health maintenance organizations (HMOs):

They have a prospective payment system.
This is a hallmark of an HMO. Members pay a predetermined premium, which covers all services provided by the HMO. Depending on the plan's coverage, with each health provider visit the member is responsible for a co-payment, usually $5 to $15.

They are a new model of managed care.
HMOs are the oldest models of managed care, some being in existence since the 1930s.

Billing paperwork remains an expensive part of the services.
Because members get all health care through one agency, it is paper-free as far as the billing goes. Co-payments are accepted at the point of service, and there are no other costs for members.

About 5% of the U.S. population is enrolled in HMOs.
Between government HMOs, such as Medicare, and private ones, such as Kaiser Permanente, over 130 million Americans—or about 45% of the country's population—use an HMO.

2. The following is true about Medicare:

Medicare is a federal health insurance program for the elderly and disabled others.
Medicare is a federal health insurance program and covers citizens and some legal aliens who are over 65 years old. It also covers people with permanent disabilities or chronic renal disease, at any age.

Medicare has two parts—A and B—and each has a monthly premium.
Medicare does have two parts. Part A covers hospital benefits and has no monthly premium. Part B is optional, covers health care provider visits, and has a monthly premium (about $50) that comes out of an elder's Social Security check.

Medicare is comprehensive and covers most of the recipient's health care costs.
Many health care needs are not covered by Medicare. It generally covers about 50% of health care costs. Clients should be encouraged to purchase a gap-filler policy, which takes care of another 25% to 35% of costs.

Medicare covers about 25% of the U.S. population.
It covers about 39 million people, or 16% of the population.

3. The following is true about Medicaid:

Medicaid is administered by each state.
Medicaid monies come to the states from the federal government. Each state determines who will receive what kinds of health care services. This makes it a uniquely different program in each state.

Medicaid has a monthly fee that recipients must pay.
Medicaid is a free program available to individuals on the basis of financial need and legal residency status.

Medicaid does not cover preventative services.
Medicaid has a major focus on preventative services, namely, infant, childhood and elder immunization programs.

Medicaid eligibility is determined by age and sex.
Eligibility is determined on the basis of financial need and residency status.

4. Health care economics as a concern for a community health nurse is:

Important to the practice setting and for agency survival

At the local level (the community health nurse and the employing agency) health care economics is very important for survival. Resourceful use of time, talent, and materials will ensure that the services will be able to continue and that the agency stays viable.

Mainly of utmost importance to the inservice educator in an agency

Health care economics should be important to all agency employees. Each in his or her own way contributes to keeping costs down, and it is not more important for any particular employee.

New and confusing and an issue for those in organizational management

The details of various insurance programs and benefits can be confusing, but it is important for community health nurses to be familiar with the basics so they can assist clients with questions they may have. Health care economics is an issue of all employees, not just those in organizational management.

Something foreign and best left to other members of the health care team

It may be foreign to community health nurses, but it is something they must become familiar with and not left to other health care team members. Client questions must be answered or referred to others if unclear.

5. Managed competition is a market-based solution to resolve the health care crisis. Ideally, it should:

Promote quality of care while keeping costs down

This is the hope of managed competition. It would combine market competition to achieve cost savings with government regulation to achieve expanded coverage.

Eliminate burdensome government regulations

Federal, state, and local regulations would continue to stay in effect to protect the consumer.

Diminish state and federal control over health care delivery

State and federal levels of government do not control health care delivery, and regulations would stay intact under managed competition.

Keep insurance companies out of the health care crisis issue

Insurance companies become more involved under managed competition, and through government regulations clients would be protected from unscrupulous practices.

ESSAY QUESTIONS

1. You have the power to finance our health system with the amount of money currently available. Give examples of changes you would make. How would these changes be managed with the finances you would have available? What services currently funded would you cut back, eliminate, or expand? How would you pay for the changes you would make?

2. Compare and contrast the services of a private physician and an HMO. Which do you prefer? Why?

INDIVIDUAL OR GROUP PROJECTS

1. Suggest that the students write, e-mail, or visit their congressperson regarding a health care financing issue.

2. Have groups of students work on Essay Question number 1 as a group project.

UNIT II

Tools of Community Health Nursing

CHAPTER 8

Communication, Collaboration, and Contracting

LEARNING OBJECTIVES

Upon mastery of this chapter, you should be able to:

- Identify the seven basic parts of the communication process.

- Describe four barriers to effective communication in community health nursing and how to deal with them.

- Explain three sets of skills necessary for effective communication in community health nursing.

- Discuss four techniques for enhancing group decision-making.

- Describe five characteristics of collaboration in community health.

- Compare the three phases common to the collaboration process.

- Identify four features of contracting in community health nursing.

- Discuss the value of contracting to both clients and community health nurses.

- Design an aggregate level contract useful in community health nursing.

KEY TERMS

Active listening	Feedback loop
Brainstorming	Formal contracting
Channel	Informal contracting
Collaboration	Message
Communication	Nominal group technique
Contracting	Nonverbal messages
Critical pathway	Nursing informatics
Decoding	Paraphrasing
Delphi technique	Receiver
Electronic meetings	Sender
Empathy	Verbal messages
Encoding	

■ Teaching Strategies

CLASSROOM TEACHING STRATEGIES

1. Bring examples of formal contracts that have been used by a community health nurse or prepare several samples of your own. Ask students to review the contracts and then evaluate the terms spelled out in the agreements.

2. Ask for student volunteers to role-play a nurse–client (family) situation. One of the student volunteers should be selected by the group to play the role of a community health nurse. The remaining students should decide which family member roles they want to act out. The community health nurse's assignment will be to negotiate an informal contract with the family. The contract could be related to one of the following issues: weight management, compliance with a medical regimen, or hygiene practices. The class as a whole will then critique the role-playing situation in relation to the contracting process and the communication skills and tools used.

CLINICAL LABORATORY TEACHING STRATEGIES

1. Assign the students to observe a community health nurse in a practice setting. Have the students identify the communication skills and the collaborative process used. The students should record their analysis of the situation in a journal and perhaps discuss their observations during a clinical post-conference. (This may be part of an observational experience to meet some other clinical laboratory objectives.)

2. Suggest that students select a client from their clinical laboratory practice setting and negotiate a formal or informal contract. This exercise may be simulated or, if appropriate, actually carried out. Ask students to share with peers the events that took place during the contracting process.

3. Suggest that the clinical laboratory students attend a variety of meetings of community members involved with health, education, or welfare issues among families you serve. Such meetings as a board meeting of a neighborhood center, a student-study team at a school, or a parent-teacher work group are good examples of experiences. Have the students observe the interactions of the members and be able to give examples of when the group members were communicating, cooperating, or collaborating. How can one tell the difference? What suggestions might each student have for the group members to reach the higher level—collaboration?

ACTIVITIES TO PROMOTE CRITICAL THINKING IN THE CLASSROOM

1. Ask the students to identify some examples of "selective perception" they have experienced with clients and discuss with fellow classmates how they dealt with the situation. Selective perception is discussed in the textbook on page 138.

2. Suggest that two students role play a difficult home visit (language barriers, noisy children in the home, adults coming and going in the house, a client who is hard of hearing, etc.), and have the rest of the class observe the "nurse" practice active listening. At the end of the role play, have the "nurse" describe how she or he applied active listening skills. Allow classmates to share their observations and give suggestions to the actors.

3. Practice the nominal group technique in class (page 142 in the textbook) using a subject of interest or a "burning issue" in the clinical laboratory site, university, or nursing department.

4. Provide a list of well-functioning collaborative groups that you are aware of in the community and have small groups of students observe one of the groups' meetings. Offer this exercise early in the term so that everyone has a chance to attend a meeting (sometimes such groups meet only monthly). Discuss their observations near the last third of the term. How well did the group members integrate the five characteristics of collaboration (pages 143–144 in the textbook)?

5. Have the students share examples of how they have been contracting with client groups—individuals, families, or aggregates. Are they formal or informal in nature? Do the students find that the contract helps the nurse–client relationship and achieve client goals?

6. Show on an overhead transparency some of the sample contracts students have used in past terms or within the current group of students. Have students take ideas from them and develop a sample contract they might use with a client group they are currently serving.

7. Have the students share the implementation of this exercise to become a good listener. Ask: has it been effective; has their circle of friends changed; do they enjoy their peer group more?

8. Follow the steps in the textbook on pages 149 to 150 to implement this activity in class. This will serve two purposes: It will assure you that the students know how to use the technique with client groups in the community, and it will improve their powers of communication.

■ Evaluation Strategies

MULTIPLE-CHOICE QUESTIONS

1. The communication process has seven parts. An important one is:

   A feedback loop
   This is the most important part of the communication process. Without feedback the process is not complete.

   Setting limits on conversations
   This is not a normal part of the communication process.

   Being goal-directed
   This might be appropriate in some conversations but is not a usual part of the communication process.

   A time limit
   This might be appropriate in some conversations but is not a usual part of the communication process.

2. Barriers to effective communication, as mentioned in this chapter, include:

   Selective perception on the part of the nurse or client
   Selective perception destroys the intent of the original message, whether it is the client or the nurse who has selective perception.

   Sharing complete and accurate information with the recipient
   This is not a barrier to effective communication. It is the goal of all communication.

The clients' use of medical terminology in conversations
This is not a barrier. It is a helpful skill.

Taking people's differences into account during communication
This is not a barrier. It is a helpful behavior.

3. Collaboration is distinguished from other types of interaction by:

Focusing on shared goals and mutual participation
Shared goals and mutual participation are distinguishing factors of collaboration.

Always including a client within the team
Clients may or may not be on the team. It depends on the nature of the collaboration whether clients are included or not.

Lengthening the time needed to meet goals
Time to accomplish tasks may or may not change when involved in collaboration.

Including flexible boundaries and responsibilities
Each person involved in a collaborative effort has defined boundaries and responsibilities.

4. The group decision-making technique of brainstorming includes:

Sharing all ideas and suggestions before discussion begins
This is how brainstorming differs from other forms of communication; all ideas are encouraged and shared.

Discussion after the generation of each new idea
Discussion occurs only after all ideas are shared in brainstorming.

Ongoing constructive criticism offered by the leader
No feedback is offered by the leader until all ideas are generated, and then all participants offer feedback.

Alternating ideas and suggestions with feedback and criticism
This is how a typical discussion or problem-solving session would work; it is not the format when a group is using the brainstorming technique.

5. Benefits of contracting with clients include:

Fostering client participation in the decision-making process
The nurse and the client contribute to the formulation of the contract, thus fostering client participation in decisions regarding the direction and activities within the contract.

Contributing to a trusting nurse–client relationship
The contract alone will not contribute to a trusting relationship. The nurse earns this trust by following through on contracted activities.

Decreasing client stress during home visits
The nurse–client contract does not in and of itself reduce or cause client stress during home visits. There should be minimal stress during home visits, unless clients do not want the nurse to visit and have not said so or if they have not been upholding their part of the contract. Either may cause stress.

Reducing client visit time by over 50%
Reducing home visit time is not the purpose of contracting. However, it might be a bit shortened because the client and nurse stay focused on the contracted items, or it could be longer because the nurse and client are engaged in actively working on contracted items.

ESSAY QUESTIONS

1. Select a group decision-making technique and identify how this technique will help solve the following two problems: (1) services being offered to prenatal clients in your agency are not well attended, and (2) agency employees are unhappy about the way vacation dates are determined.

2. Provide an example of a formal contract and suggest how the community health nurse could present the idea in the following examples: (1) a family has a history of obesity and wants to change this pattern, (2) a group of seniors at a local senior center would like a community health nurse to provide health information classes on a regular basis, and (3) your agency and a pharmaceutical company are collaborating on testing a new osmotic product on selected clients.

INDIVIDUAL OR GROUP PROJECTS

1. Collect samples of contracts used in a variety of settings with different groups of clients. Compare and contrast the contracts. Select parts of each contract that appeal to you the most in order to develop model contracts for future use.

2. With a group of peers, participate in a variety of role-playing scenarios that demonstrate core communications skills, barriers to effective communication, and collaboration. "Contract" with the faculty member to demonstrate these techniques as part of your course grade.

CHAPTER 9

Health Promotion Through Education

Learning Objectives

Upon mastery of this chapter, you should be able to:

- Identify how the nurse collaborates with other professionals, using *Healthy People 2010* as a guide for educational and community-based programs.

- Describe the community health nurse's role as educator in promoting health and preventing or postponing morbidity.

- Identify educational activities for the nurse to use that are appropriate for each of the three domains of learning.

- Select learning theories that are applicable to an individual, family, or aggregate client.

- Identify health teaching models to use when planning health education activities.

- Select teaching methods and materials that facilitate learning for clients at different developmental levels.

- Develop teaching plans focusing on primary, secondary, and tertiary levels of prevention for clients of all ages.

- Identify teaching strategies for the community health nurse to use when encountering clients with special learning needs.

- Locate appropriate multimedia resources to enhance client learning.

KEY TERMS

Accommodation (Piaget)
Adaptation (Piaget)
Affective domain
Anticipatory guidance
Assimilation (Piaget)
Cognitive domain

Gestalt-field
Learning
Operationalize
Psychomotor domain
Teaching

■ Teaching Strategies

CLASSROOM TEACHING STRATEGIES

1. Have students select and provide rationale for using a learning theory that is applicable to an individual, family, or aggregate for each of the following scenarios: a young mother in need of enhanced parenting skills; an intergenerational family of seven members who have a terminally ill member being cared for at home; and an aggregate of preschool-aged children needing a class on personal hygiene.

2. Following your lecture on the seven teaching-learning principles, ask students to identify how they were used in the presentation.

3. Ask students to select teaching methods and materials that would be appropriate in the three scenarios presented in classroom strategy number 1.

CLINICAL LABORATORY TEACHING STRATEGIES

1. Each student should select a teaching project to implement with a group of his or her choice in the community. Each student should submit a formal teaching plan that includes the name of the group being taught, contact person (schoolteacher, senior center director, etc.), teaching topic, evidence of learner readiness (cognitive level, age level, interest), behavioral objectives, outline of content, methods and materials used (include rationale and resources needed), and evaluation strategies (of the client's knowledge of the subject and one of your teaching style completed by the students). To enhance the teacher role, suggest students teach the same content to extremely different age groups so the student can identify different depths of content (perhaps knowledge level for first graders versus application level for high school students, and synthesis for adults), methods and materials (puppets for 5-year-olds, a video for junior high

students, a discussion for adults), and evaluation strategies (verbal questions and answer sessions for preschoolers and older adults or a pencil-and-paper evaluation tool for 6th graders).

2. Each student should present 10 minutes of the plan he or she created (in Clinical Laboratory Strategies number 1) to his or her peers during a clinical conference. The peers should "behave" like the intended learners might (preschoolers, junior high school students, seniors, etc.). After the presentation, the other students and instructor should verbally critique the sample of teaching and give positive and constructive feedback that will enhance the teaching with the intended learners.

3. Have the students implement the teaching plan with the intended learners with the instructor in attendance. After the teaching session, give verbal and written feedback for student growth in the community health nursing role of teacher.

ACTIVITIES TO PROMOTE CRITICAL THINKING IN THE CLASSROOM

1. Facilitate a general discussion of individual student learning styles. Use this information to ask what teaching methods they use with client groups that consider the possible learning styles of clients.

2. Ask the students to identify the potential recipients of health teaching and possible learning needs among the following selected groups:

   a. Seniors living in a mobile home park

   b. Employees in a medical laboratory of a large clinic

   c. Parents of pre-schoolers attending an enrichment program 2 mornings a week

   d. Pregnant teens attending a local high school

   e. A group of boys working on Boy Scout health and safety badges

3. Through your connections in the community and understanding of the importance of community leaders being knowledgeable regarding health care issues that affect the local community, establish an ongoing inservice program, using students as the teachers, to educate political staff members on health-related issues that focus on public health principles.

4. Discuss the types of teaching projects the students are implementing with clients in their clinical laboratory experiences. Do they focus on cognitive, affective, or psychomotor skills? Discuss ways to enhance cognitive-focused teaching by including affective learning activities. Do the same with psychomotor skills and affective learning activities. Review the student teaching plans for this inclusion. Ask students whether the inclusion leads to any noticeable changes in client learning. How do they know? What did they observe that was different?

5. Have the students practice using the verbs given on page 167 in the textbook to develop measurable behavioral objectives as they work in small groups designing a flyer for a hypothetical health fair for elementary school children, high school students, community members visiting a mall, and seniors gathering for a Dixieland jazz festival.

6. Discuss the various teaching models presented in the textbook on pages 159 to 162. Suggest that groups of students use different ones and report back in 2 or 3 weeks how they used this model to guide the development of their teaching topic and with what group it was used.

7. Select several peers whom you admire as role model teachers. Ask them to come to your class and present a short demonstration of their teaching style (they may teach something very different from nursing). Allow time for questions and answers regarding the role model's development of her or his teaching methods.

   Another possibility is to use community speakers you have gotten to know and have them present pertinent community health nursing information in lieu of your lecture; choose them for their skillful teaching styles in addition to the content they have to share. After the guest has left, ask the students what about the presentation they most enjoyed and learned from. Suggest they emulate the methods and styles used in their next teaching experience.

8. Have the students share negative teaching experiences they have encountered, either as a student or as the teacher. Ask students the following questions: How was the negative situation resolved? Was it addressed constructively, or was it ignored and allowed to continue? What would you do now to prevent, limit, or stop such an experience the next time?

9. Suggest that each student participate in this activity early in the term. About halfway through the term, have the students bring the assortment of pamphlets and brochures to class and put them on display for all students to see. Allow class time for the students to copy addresses, phone numbers, Internet addresses, and e-mail addresses of sources they would want to contact.

■ Evaluation Strategies

MULTIPLE-CHOICE QUESTIONS

1. The following example demonstrates the knowledge level of cognitive learning. After attending the nurse's class on nutrition, the client:

   Can name three foods high in iron
   This is an example of the knowledge level of learning, the first level of cognitive learning.

   Compares the nutrient value in foods
   This is an example of the analysis level of learning, the fourth level of cognitive learning.

   Eats well-balanced meals
   This is an example of the application level of learning, the third level of cognitive learning.

   Plans recipes that are low in fat
   This is an example of the synthesis level of learning, the fifth level of cognitive learning.

2. The following example demonstrates the application level of cognitive learning. After attending the nurse's class on nutrition, the client:

   Eats well-balanced meals
   This is an example of the application level of learning, the third level of cognitive learning.

   Can name three foods high in iron
   This is an example of the knowledge level of learning, the first level of cognitive learning.

   Compares the nutrient value in food
   This is an example of the analysis level of learning, the fourth level of cognitive learning.

   Plans recipes that are low in fat
   This is an example of the synthesis level of learning, the fifth level of cognitive learning.

3. A community health nurse is using behavioral theory when the teaching focuses on:

   Changes in response to a stimulus
   Behavioral theory is grounded in stimulus-response behaviors, and changes occur in response to a stimuli. Skinner and Pavlov were famous behavioral theorists.

   Meeting a hierarchy of needs
   This is based on Maslow's Hierarchy of Needs and is a humanistic theory. In humanistic theory there is a belief that there is a natural tendency for people to learn.

   The learners and their self-confidence and personal mastery
   This is characteristic of social learning theory. Bandura is an important social learning theorist.

   A person's natural tendency to learn
   In humanistic theory there is a natural tendency for people to learn. They do so in an encouraging environment.

4. A community health nurse works with a new mother to teach her how to give her infant a bath. After the nurse demonstrates how to safely hold the newborn and use a washcloth and baby soap, the new mother completes the baby's bath herself with the nurse observing and offering encouraging comments. The new mother is demonstrating an example of the following domain of learning:

   Psychomotor
   In the psychomotor domain the learner demonstrates a newly learned skill with the nurse offering guidance and positive reinforcement. This is what the new mother is demonstrating to the nurse.

   Cognitive
   The learner demonstrates learning that involves the mind and thinking processes, grasping the meaning and relationship of a series of facts.

   Affective
   The learning occurring in the affective domain includes emotions, feelings, or affect.

   Social
   There is no learning domain referred to as social. However, learning takes place in a social context.

5. Veronica Sommers is 32 years old, a wife and mother of two children, and was a bank manager before coming to the nursing program. She is finishing a baccalaureate nursing program in a few months. She learns best when she can plan and carry out her own learning activities, uses past experiences to help with current learning, and applies learning immediately. The learning theory that would best fit Veronica's learning style is:

   Knowles' adult learning theory
   Veronica's behaviors support the tenets of Knowles' adult learning theory. She is a self-directed learner, experienced, ready to learn, and is problem centered rather than theoretically oriented. (A note to faculty: Adult students often respond best when faculty use Knowles' adult learning theory. However, adult learners are open to theoretical support for nursing actions, but they are anxious for the actions to come first. This often goes against teaching principles of theory first, then practice. They do best when clinical laboratory experiences are tied tightly to the theory and do not lag far behind the theory.)

Bandura's social learning theory
In social learning theory the aim is to explain behavior and facilitate learning. This is not supported by the description of Veronica's learning style.

The Gestalt-Field family of theories
In this theory it is assumed that people are neither good nor bad, but that they simply interact with their environment and their learning is related to perception. This is not supported by the description of Veronica's learning style.

Maslow's Hierarchy of Needs theory
This theory suggests that there is a leveling of needs among people, and lower levels (safety and security) must be met before higher levels (self-esteem and self-worth) are met. This is not supported by the description of Veronica's learning style.

6. A community health nursing student is planning to teach a group of 20 preschool children about dental health. Based on what he knows about 4-year-olds, their physical and cognitive abilities, and teaching principles, which of the following activities would be most appropriate during the teaching session?

Have the students practice "brushing" with their finger and "make-believe" toothpaste
Twenty 4-year-old children can be overwhelming to a novice teacher. It is best to keep them in their seats or places on the floor. The nurse will have better classroom control, psychomotor skills can be observed, preschoolers enjoy "make believe," and time and resources are conserved.

Have the children brush their teeth in the sink in the bathroom down the hall from the classroom.
The class may get out of control. Twenty children cannot be supervised at the same time in the bathroom, and who will be supervising the rest of the children (and what will they be doing?) while three or four are brushing their teeth? What if a child is allergic to the toothpaste? If the nursing student has gotten samples of toothbrushes and toothpaste, it is best that the classroom teacher give them to the students as they leave for home with instructions not to open the packages until their parents see their "gift."

Have each of the children eat a candy bar and then show one another how "dirty" their teeth get.
The class may get out of control. Twenty 4-year-old children eating candy bars can get quite messy. What if a child is allergic to chocolate or nuts or is not allowed to eat candy? It is best to give any food gifts to the teacher to decide how they are

to be distributed and use a different way to demonstrate "dirty" teeth. Smear a soft chocolate bar on a stuffed animal's teeth or on a picture of a popular TV character—4-year-olds will enjoy oohing and aahing over this "funny" (and less messy) example.

Bring a variety of "teeth healthy" snacks for the children to eat and discuss why they are better for their teeth than other snacks.
The class may get out of control. Twenty 4-year-old children eating even healthy snacks can get quite messy. What if a child is allergic to a certain fruit or wheat in a cracker or is not allowed to eat between meals? It is best to give any food gifts to the teacher to decide how they are to be distributed and use a different way to demonstrate healthy snacks. Hold up pictures of people eating healthy snacks versus unhealthy snacks and have them shout loudly which one is the healthy snack (4 year olds will enjoy having permission to make a lot of noise while in the preschool classroom, something they ordinarily may not be allowed to do).

7. A student nurse is developing a class in low-sodium foods for a group of 20 senior citizens at the senior center. She wants to impress the elders with the amount of sodium in some foods versus others. The best teaching method with these elders includes:

Find out some of the usual food items eaten, have the products at the senior center, discuss the nutritional information panel on each product, and allow the attendees to suggest alternatives if the product is high in sodium.
This uses fewer resources than other methods, yet it includes the seniors in an active teaching/learning method. It does not put any seniors at risk (eating sodium-laden foods) or on the spot (did not bring a food item to the center today).

Have the seniors bring a food item to the center and have each person taste the foods. Have them judge how much sodium is in each product and follow the activity with a discussion.
This uses the seniors' resources and may put a senior on the spot (did not bring a food item to the center today). It also puts some seniors at risk (eating sodium-laden foods). However, it is an active teaching/learning method and may be a good method with a younger and healthy population.

Hold up pictures of foods high and low in sodium and tell why one product would be better than another. The seniors could take copies of the information home with them at the end of the teaching session.

This is a very passive teaching style; it could get boring and lose the audience's interest. Can the seniors see well enough to appreciate the pictures? This is not the best choice.

Show a video of cooking without sodium and follow it with a discussion of foods to eat and foods to avoid.

To use this method the student nurse would have to know the audience, facility, and its resources well. Will the room accommodate everyone seeing and hearing the video? Is the screen going to be big enough for everyone to see? What if the group is large? Do all people in the group do their own cooking? It is not the best choice with the information given in this question.

ESSAY QUESTIONS

1. Select one topic to teach (nutrition, safety, exercise, etc.) and adapt it to preschoolers and senior citizens. Identify the appropriate learning objectives, methods and materials, and evaluation methods for each group. Include the rationale for the differences you select.

2. Write a behavioral objective at each of the six levels of cognitive learning for a selected topic.

3. You are teaching a group of people attending a clinic in the community about beginning to feed infants table food. The participants are various ages, male and female, come from a variety of cultures, and have different educational levels. Identify factors you must consider before you begin teaching, and give the rationale for these considerations.

INDIVIDUAL OR GROUP PROJECTS

1. Have small groups of students develop behavioral objectives at different levels of cognitive learning for several different topics. Write them down for all to see. Have the students critique them for measurability and appropriateness.

2. Observe a community health nurse teaching a group of clients and critique her or his effectiveness. What suggestions might you give the nurse? What behaviors might you like to incorporate into your own teaching style?

CHAPTER 10

The Community Health Nurse as Leader, Change Agent, and Case Manager

LEARNING OBJECTIVES

Upon mastery of this chapter, you should be able to:

- Describe three characteristics of leadership.
- Summarize five leadership theories.
- Compare and contrast five leadership styles.
- Describe five leadership functions.
- Differentiate between four power bases and four power sources.
- Discuss the concept of empowerment and its significance for community health nursing.
- Explain the three stages of change.
- Discuss the eight steps in planned change.
- Identify three planned change strategies.
- Summarize six principles for effecting change in community health.
- Describe the case-management role of the community health nurse.

KEY TERMS

Autocratic leadership style	Planned change
Autonomous leadership style	Power
Case management	Power bases
Change	Power-coercive change
Empirical-rational change	strategy
strategy	Power sources
Empowerment	Revolutionary change
Evolutionary change	Stages of change
Force field analysis	Transactional leadership
Leadership	style
Normative-reeducative	Transformational
change strategy	leadership style
Participative leadership style	

■ Teaching Strategies

CLASSROOM TEACHING STRATEGIES

1. Prior to the class on Chapter 10 content, have the students respond in writing to the following questions. (The responses should be confidential, but ask for volunteers to discuss their responses.)

   a. Who is the most effective person or best leader you have personally known?

   b. What are his or her major characteristics?

   c. Describe the worst leader you have ever personally known.

   d. What makes the leader so bad?

2. Think of a community health nurse who is an effective leader. Ask the nurse to speak to the class about situations she or he has encountered in her or his role as a leader and change agent.

CLINICAL LABORATORY TEACHING STRATEGIES

1. Assign the students to identify forces in the health care delivery system locally, regionally, or nationally that they would like to change. Ask them to identify forces that may inhibit change and discuss how they, as change agents, would facilitate the change process.

2. Assign the students to interview a well-known community leader (mayor, religious leader, etc.). Questions the students might ask include the following:

   a. What are your present concerns for the community?

   b. What are your visions for the future?

   c. How do you view your role as a community leader?

   d. What obstacles have you encountered when acting as a change agent?

   e. How would you describe your leadership style?

ACTIVITIES TO PROMOTE CRITICAL THINKING IN THE CLASSROOM

1. Rather than doing this activity as an exercise, actually plan a health fair for the local community as a whole or an aggregate in the community, such as teens, elders, or employees of a large company. Use steps a to i as a planning guide.

2. Use this exercise in the class to identify valuable leadership skills as determined by the students. The exercise can then be used with client groups in the community. In addition, invite local community health agency nursing leaders to speak to the class and ask each to identify leadership skills important for beginning community health nurses to have if thinking of employment in public health.

■ Evaluation Strategies

MULTIPLE-CHOICE QUESTIONS

1. Lewin's three-stage change model follows this pattern:

   Unfreeze, change, refreeze
   In Lewin's change model there are three steps: unfreezing the old behavior, implementing the change, and then refreezing the new change in place to integrate it into the system.

   Unfreeze, plan, integrate
   These are not the three stages of Lewin's change model.

   Plan, organize, coordinate
   These are not the three stages of Lewin's change model.

   Plan, relearn, integrate
   These are not the three stages of Lewin's change model.

2. The normative-reductive strategy of change assumes that:

   Information alone is not enough, and behaviors change through persuasion.
   Normative-reductive strategies not only give information but also directly influence people to change attitudes and behaviors through persuasion.

   Compliance by the client system will occur through the use of power to effect change.
   This describes the power-coercive change strategy. Coercion is based on fear to effect change, and the change agents derive power from the law, position, a group, or personal power such as charisma.

   People are rational and will adopt a new practice because it is in their best interest.
   This describes the empirical-rational change strategy. When people are presented with empirical information, they will change because they are rational and will do what is in their best interest.

   A participative leadership style will be used.
   The normative-reductive strategy of change is different from leadership styles. During a change process there will be a variety of people who use different leadership styles.

3. If a community health nursing leader uses an autocratic leadership style, she or he:

   Uses the power of the position to influence followers
   The autocratic leadership style uses the power of the position to influence followers. Autocratic leaders give orders and expects followers to obey based on the power of her or his position.

   Involves followers in the decision-making process
   This describes the democratic participative leadership style. These types of leaders are people oriented and focus on relationships and teamwork.

   Is facilitative and encourages independence among group members
   This describes the autonomous leadership style. The leader's role is to set general parameters and to facilitate followers' progress.

   Encourages the use of magnetic and inspirational personality and behaviors
   This describes the charismatic theory of leadership. These leaders lead by getting an emotional commitment from the followers and arousing strong feelings of loyalty and enthusiasm.

4. If a community health nursing leader uses the participative leadership style, she or he:

   Involves followers in the decision-making process
   This describes the participative leadership style, which is democratic. These types of leaders are people oriented and focus on relationships and teamwork.

   Is facilitative and encourages independence among group members
   This describes the autonomous leadership style. The leader's role is to set general parameters and to facilitate followers' progress.

Encourages the use of magnetic and inspirational personality and behaviors.

This describes the charismatic theory of leadership. These leaders lead by getting an emotional commitment from the followers and arousing strong feelings of loyalty and enthusiasm.

Uses the power of the position to influence followers

The autocratic leadership style uses the power of the position to influence followers. Autocratic leaders give orders and expect followers to obey based on the power of her or his position.

5. Debbie Taylor is a fairly new graduate nurse. After 6 months of working as a community health nurse, she was promoted to team leader. People say she is a natural leader. She has a desire to lead, is ambitious and full of energy, intelligent, and has self-confidence. Which of the following theories does it sound like Debbie models?

Trait theory

This is the "great man" theory, which contends that a few people are born with the traits necessary to be a great leader and they possess certain specific personality qualities, or traits, that make them leaders, such as displayed by Debbie Taylor.

Behavioral theory

This theory proposes that the success of a leader depends on the leader's behavior rather than his or her personality traits.

Contingency theory

This theory describes leadership in terms of the leader's ability to adapt to the situation, and success is contingent on the situation encountered by the leader.

Charismatic theory

According to this theory, leadership occurs because of a magnetic and inspirational personality and behavior.

6. Jonathan Wiley is a supervising community health nurse. He often has meetings with his staff and influences them to change beliefs and actions through convincing discussions he leads. This form of power is referred to as:

Persuasive power

This is the type of power Jonathan is using. He has the power to persuade his team members and influence their way of thinking and acting in relation to work.

Reward power

A leader using reward power has the ability to influence people by granting rewards that they view as valuable, such as bonus pay, time off, or a particular case assignment.

Coercive power

A leader using coercive power forces compliance based on fear. The team members comply with orders if they believe that not doing so would result in a penalty.

Information power

A leader using information power uses his or her access to or possession of valued information to influence others. Knowledge is power.

7. Case management is a model used by community health nurses for decades. Characteristics basic to case management include:

Interdisciplinary collaboration

The case manager role cannot be accomplished without interdisciplinary collaboration as the role includes working with professionals and paraprofessionals from a variety of health and social agencies, in addition to the client.

Autonomous practice

The community health nurse as a case manager works with many other people in professional and paraprofessional positions.

Resistance to change

Being able to initiate or participate in change is necessary as a successful case manager. Resisting change is not.

Enhancing restraining forces

Restraining forces are the negative forces inhibiting change. These are not to be enhanced, and change in and of itself is a different issue from case management.

ESSAY QUESTIONS

1. Describe the attributes an ideal leader should have in the role of director of nursing in a community health nursing agency.

2. Briefly describe your leadership style. What aspects of your style would you like to enhance or change?

INDIVIDUAL OR GROUP PROJECTS

1. Perhaps several students are working on a group project in some class they are taking or organization they belong to. Suggest they examine the leadership style of the group leader. Have the students answer the following questions: What does the leader do right and wrong? What leadership style does the leader display? How would you lead the group differently?

2. Complete a group project using the Activities to Promote Critical Thinking at the end of Chapter 10 in the textbook.

CHAPTER 11

Research in Community Health Nursing

LEARNING OBJECTIVES

Upon mastery of this chapter, you should be able to:

- Explain the difference between quantitative research and qualitative research.

- Describe the eight steps of the research process.

- Differentiate between experimental and nonexperimental research design.

- Analyze the potential impact of research on community health nursing practice.

- Evaluate the application of a community-based research study.

- Identify the community health nurse's role in conducting research and using research findings.

KEY TERMS

Conceptual model	Nonexperimental design
Control group	Qualitative research
Descriptive statistics	Quantitative research
Experimental design	Quasi-experiment
Experimental group	Randomization
Generalizability	Reliability
Inferential statistics	Research
Instrument	True experiment
Meta-analysis	Validit

■ Teaching Strategies

CLASSROOM TEACHING STRATEGIES

1. Arrange for nurses who are working in the community, or at the university and participating in research, to speak to the class about their research activities. Encourage them to discuss both successes and pitfalls associated with their efforts.

2. Assign students to bring to class community health nursing research articles from current (within the last 5 years) nursing journals. Each student should select or be assigned a specific topic of interest (such as AIDS, stress reduction, battered spouses,

health promotion, etc.). Use the journal articles to discuss the steps of the research process and the role of the community health nurse in conducting research.

CLINICAL LABORATORY TEACHING STRATEGIES

1. Have the students identify an area of interest specific to their clinical laboratory setting that could be the focus of a community health nursing investigation. At a clinical conference, ask the students to describe how an investigation could be conducted and what impact such a study would have on community health nursing practice locally. Recommend that students share their research ideas with staff members, if appropriate. If there is interest and an avenue of financial support for such research, include students in the study, if feasible.

2. Ask the students to discuss with agency personnel research activities in which these individuals are participating or have participated and their plans for future study. Have students share this information during a clinical conference or in their clinical laboratory journals.

ACTIVITIES TO PROMOTE CRITICAL THINKING IN THE CLASSROOM

1. Use similar examples from your local community to develop additional research questions. Allow students to share some of their observations in the community and develop research questions from their clinical laboratory experience.

2. Have the students select high-risk groups from their clinical laboratory experiences and determine whether the groups would be receptive to an educational program to reduce their risk. Suggest that the students formulate a research question, describe a conceptual framework they might use in this study, and have them defend their choices.

3. Repeat the exercise in this question using a new community health research in the literature or a recent study conducted by faculty or graduate students in your nursing program. How might the outcomes impact health policy or community health nursing practice?

4. Facilitate a general discussion regarding community health nursing's responsibility in disseminating research information to colleagues and other community health professionals.

5. Suggest that the students bring to class their findings from the Internet on the most current and effective forms of treatment for TB. Apply this information to hypothetically implement new approaches with your specific target population. You could replicate this exercise using any current issue of concern to high-risk clients in your community.

▪ Evaluation Strategies

MULTIPLE-CHOICE QUESTIONS

1. The function of a conceptual model for a research study is to:

   Clarify the focus and direction of the study
   The conceptual model clarifies the focus and direction of the study and looks at the world in terms of nursing major concerns.

   Provide evidence that an instrument is valid
   The conceptual model does not include the data-gathering instrument. Thus, it cannot provide evidence of its validity.

   Limit the breadth and depth of the study
   Although the conceptual model provides the structure and framework of the study, the researcher has to decide how deep and broad the study will ultimately be in the number of research questions and size of the population used.

   Enhance the possibility of relating findings to other populations
   This is not the function of the conceptual model. Size of the study is the main factor in relating the findings to other populations.

2. Inferential statistics may be used to analyze data. This form of statistical analysis:

   Implies that relationships found in the group studied can be generalized to a larger group
   Inferential studies are used to imply that relationships seen in the group of individuals

studied (sample) are likely to exist in the larger group of concern (population).

   Implies that the data collected are appropriate and valuable and can be analyzed
   In general, there is no guarantee of appropriateness or value of data. Specifically, the purpose of using inferential statistics is not to guarantee that data are appropriate or valuable.

   Permits the investigator to initiate a preliminary investigation of subjects
   This describes a pilot study. Inferential statistics used in analysis are not involved in preliminary investigation, or a pilot study.

   Describes the data collected in an organized manner according to defined variables
   This is not how inferential statistics are used. It describes the analysis of collected data.

3. An experimental design requires that the investigator:

   Manipulates one of the variables
   A true experimental study is characterized by manipulation of one of the variables, randomization, and the use of a control group.

   Non-randomly assign subjects to groups
   A true experimental study is characterized by randomizing the study.

   Control all variables without manipulation
   In a true experimental study it is important to control one of the variables, not all of the variables.

   Balance the study by having four different groups in it
   It is only necessary to have two groups—the randomized study group and the randomized control group. In some large studies there may be three or more different groups.

4. Judy Phillips, a community health nurse, is prepared to conduct a literature review for a research study on teenaged fatherhood. She know that this includes:

   An overview of current literature in the area, followed by an in-depth study of literature
   An overview of recent literature assists the researcher in getting direction and focus on a topic of interest. This is followed by an in-depth study of current (last 5 years) literature.

   An in-depth study of the literature in the area of interest for at least the last 20 years
   This depth of literature review is too deep and would uncover too much information to handle in a useful manner; also, some articles would be outdated. However, when doing a literature review the researcher may come across an older,

"classic" piece of literature, which can become a tremendous support for the current literature used.

Multiple sources of information, including current lay literature, historical documents, and the tabloid press

Primary sources of data from professional literature are preferred. Depending on the study, an historical document might provide a valuable piece of information. The tabloid press is not used.

No more than three to five articles that are studied in-depth and incorporated into the body of the study

A literature review should uncover professional research on the topic for the last 5 years. Selected research is incorporated into the body of the study and supported by replicated or associated studies, but there is no limit on the number of articles.

5. Judy is considering a variety of data collection sources for her study and includes:

Opinions

Opinion polls, or asking subjects for their opinions on topics, are considered valid information to gather.

Gossip

Gossip has no place in legitimate research.

Rumors

Rumors have no place in legitimate research.

Hearsay

Hearsay has no place in legitimate research.

6. Judy wants to ensure that her study is reliable. She can demonstrate reliability by:

Obtaining similar results from the instrument with the same population on two separate occasions

This "test" determines that the tool or instrument is reliable.

Assuring that an instrument measures the variables it is supposed to measure

This defines another attribute of a good research study, validity.

Randomizing the study participants when selecting study subjects

Randomization is ideal but not always practical. At time the subjects are chosen because of convenience. If it is not a true experimental design, randomization is not critical and yet the study results can still be reliable.

Making sure that the results of the study can be applied to other, similar populations

This describes generalizability. Although an ideal outcome, it is not always possible or practical to achieve.

ESSAY QUESTIONS

1. Think of a disease process or health-related issue affecting the last community health client you visited. Using the steps of the research process, design a study involving that issue. Describe a study that could be conducted in your community with resources you know are available that would focus on the issue chosen.

2. Follow the same format suggested in question 1, but select a health-related issue that you see in yourself (stress, weight, lack of organization, spirituality, etc.) and design a study with nursing students as the subjects.

INDIVIDUAL OR GROUP PROJECTS

1. Conduct a mini-literature review to find a topic that is currently an issue in the community health agency you are using for your community health nursing clinical laboratory. Find out from the administration and instructor whether you can apply the findings of the research to a portion of the population the agency serves.

2. Suggest to the staff members or administration in an agency with which you are affiliated that one or several students assist them in conducting research. As part of the course requirements, actively include yourself in the research process.

3. Assist a faculty member in current research she or he is conducting. The research steps that are especially suited for student involvement are the literature review, data collection, and communicating the findings.

Quality Measurement and Improvement in Community Health Nursing

LEARNING OBJECTIVES

Upon mastery of this chapter, you should be able to:

- Develop a working knowledge of quality improvement and management terms.

- Discuss five factors affecting quality measurement and improvement in community health nursing.

- Compare and contrast six models for measuring and improving the quality of care and their usefulness in community health nursing.

- Identify six techniques used in quality measurement and improvement in community health programs.

- Discuss the role of the nurse within quality measurement and improvement programs in community health nursing agencies.

KEY TERMS

Audit	Quality improvement
Benchmarking	Quality indicators
Concurrent review	Quality measurement
Peer review	Retrospective review
Quality assurance	Risk assessment
Quality care	Standards of care
Quality circles	Total quality management

■ Teaching Strategies

CLASSROOM TEACHING STRATEGIES

1. Ask a representative of a health care agency in the community to speak to the class about the process of quality management used in the agency. What specific quality measurement and improvement strategies do they employ? How do the nurses in the agency participate in the quality management program?

2. Examine the six models of quality management presented in this chapter and determine the one(s)

most helpful for a public agency (city health department) and private agency (a for-profit home health agency). Discuss reasons for the choices made.

CLINICAL LABORATORY TEACHING STRATEGIES

1. In the agency in which students are experiencing their community health nursing clinical laboratory practicum, ask one of the nursing administrators to discuss with the students the agency's quality management system for the nursing staff.

2. Have the students conduct a chart audit on a client they are serving, using the agency's quality management assessment tools (checklists, survey, etc.). Discuss the ease in using, time involved, benefits of using the tools, and so on. Evaluate the information gained along with the time needed to conduct the audit. What support do the students give for maintaining or changing the present system?

ACTIVITIES TO PROMOTE CRITICAL THINKING IN THE CLASSROOM

1. Using the agencies the students are placed in for their clinical laboratory experience as examples, evaluate their quality based on the characteristics of a quality community health program found on page 220. Discuss with the students what changes the agencies might make if they do not meet all the characteristics. Would the changes be feasible for the agency to accomplish? If so, would a meeting with the administrator of the agency to discuss your findings or concerns be appropriate?

2. Have the students ask the agencies used for their clinical laboratory experience whether they use a model for quality management. If they do not, do they have a set of guidelines they follow as their quality management program? Suggest the students bring a copy of either or both to class from the

various agencies and discuss them. Are they serving the purpose for which they were designed? Are they automatically and continuously used or followed only before an accreditation visit? How is the student work incorporated into the quality management program?

3. Using the same idea as in this exercise, develop standards and criteria for specific services the students provide in the agency used for their clinical laboratory experience if they are different from other professional staff. For example, the students may set up a flu-shot clinic for elders in the fall that is separate from the usual services of the agency. What standards and criteria will guide the implementation of such a service?

4. Suggest that the students use the concept of a quality circle (page 218 in the textbook) to improve an aspect of their life on campus. This might include introducing the concept in extracurricular campus groups they are members of, a fraternity or sorority they belong to, or on committees within the department of nursing.

5. Select a few current articles that address quality measurement and improvement in community health nursing. Compare and contrast the recommendations in the articles with the information found in Chapter 12 of the textbook. Use this information to enhance your lecture or student discussion on the issue of quality measurement and improvement.

■ Evaluation Strategies

MULTIPLE-CHOICE QUESTIONS

1. Facilitation of ongoing self-evaluation in the work setting is accomplished through:

   Quality indicators
   Through the use of quality indicators as a quality measurement tool to measure client outcomes or process outcomes, facilitation of ongoing self-evaluation occurs.

   Benchmarking
   Benchmarking is accomplished by studying another's processes in order to improve one's own processes.

   Use of the nursing process
   Although the nursing process helps organize care to clients, it is the quality indicators used as a quality measurement tool that facilitate ongoing self-evaluation.

Peer review
This is a system of reviewing and evaluating the quality of care given, thus focusing on the provider of care and not the outcomes.

2. The six characteristics of a quality health care program are comprehensiveness, effectiveness, acceptability, accessibility, efficiency, and provider competence. In evaluating accessibility, which of the following questions would be appropriate?

   Does the agency connect with the population served and find adequate ways to meet the public's health needs?
   Accessibility of an agency is demonstrated if it is readily involved with its population on a timely basis despite barriers that may be present.

   Do the services provided make good use of available funds?
   This describes efficiency in an agency.

   Are the nurses using the most current information and resources available?
   This describes provider competence.

   Is the population being served satisfied with the care they are receiving?
   Client satisfaction is another measure of caregiving and does not clearly measure accessibility.

3. The six characteristics of a quality health care program are comprehensiveness, effectiveness, acceptability, accessibility, efficiency, and provider competence. In evaluating efficiency, which of the following questions would be appropriate?

   Do the services provided make good use of available funds?
   This describes efficiency in an agency.

   Does the agency connect with the population served and find adequate ways to meet the public's health needs?
   Accessibility of an agency is demonstrated if it is readily involved with its population on a timely basis despite barriers that may be present.

   Are the nurses using the most current information and resources available?
   This describes provider competence.

   Is the population being served satisfied with the care they are receiving?
   Client satisfaction is another measure of caregiving and does not clearly measure accessibility.

4. A quality circle can best be described as:

A style of participative management that shares the decision-making process with staff

A quality circle includes employees in problem-solving and decision-making to enhance the quality of care to clients.

The financing of an organization from purchasing through the delivery of services

This describes the budgetary flow within an organization and does not describe a quality circle.

The parameters a nurse must consider as care is delivered

These parameters encompass the standards of care nurses follow when care is delivered.

A form of reward to an agency when it has met criteria demonstrating excellence

A quality circle is a process tool and not a reward of excellence. Having clients meet goals and achieve a higher level of wellness is a form of reward for an agency.

5. Several quality management models are helpful in measuring and improving the quality of care. They are designed differently but are developed to enhance caregiving. One has a unique feature—placing the client within the model. This is the:

Quality Health Outcomes model

The design in this model is different from the others included in the text in that it includes the client within the model.

Upwardly spiraling quality assurance feedback loop

This one is similar to the ANA quality assurance model but takes it further by adding a feedback loop.

Omaha system model

This model is comprehensive with a patient classification scheme, an intervention scheme, a supervisory shared visit tool, and a problem rating scale for outcomes. The client is not included within the model.

Hoesing and Kirk quality management model

This model is designed for supervisory and administrative personnel as well as the individual professional nurse. The client is not included within the model.

ESSAY QUESTIONS

1. Review the charting you have done on a client you have been visiting. How would you be able to measure whether quality care had been delivered to this client by reviewing your charting?

2. Identify the services that you feel should be provided by the "ideal" community health agency. Using the six techniques used in quality measurement and improvement outlined in this chapter, how would you measure success?

INDIVIDUAL OR GROUP PROJECTS

1. Ask the nurse manager of a community agency if you may participate in the chart audit process of the agency. Critique the methods used. Ask questions about the process and possibly make suggestions to improve the process in a meeting with the nursing manager.

2. Initiate a quality circle concept among a group of peers and your instructor in the community health nursing course. Use this participative management tool to evaluate class functioning based on established standards (the course objectives).

CHAPTER 13

Policy Making and Community Health Advocacy

LEARNING OBJECTIVES

Upon mastery of this chapter, you should be able to:

- Define health policy and explain how it is established.

- Analyze the influence of health policy on community health and nursing practice.

- Explain the role of special interest groups in health care reform and policy making.

- Define political empowerment and describe ways in which community health nurses can become politically empowered.

- Identify the four stages in the policy process and briefly explain what each entails.

- Explain the role of community health nurses in determining a community's health policy needs.

- Identify the 10 steps in mobilizing a community for political action.

- Describe the steps involved in how a bill becomes law.

- Explain several methods of communicating with legislators on policy issues.

- List at least four political strategies for community health nursing.

KEY TERMS

Community health advocacy	Political action
Distributive health policy	Political action committee (PAC)
Health policy	
Lobbying	Political empowerment
Polarization	Politics
Policy	Public policy
Policy analysis	Regulatory health policy
Policy system	Special interest group

■ Teaching Strategies

CLASSROOM TEACHING STRATEGIES

1. Invite a community activist to speak to the class about his or her area of political interest. Ideally the area of interest is involved with existing health policies. If possible, find a community health nurse who is involved in these issues. For example, in our community a retired nurse who served in Vietnam was instrumental in establishing the Women's Memorial in Washington, D.C. Her discussion of her efforts, along with those of other women who served in Vietnam, as they spent years involved with the federal political system was very moving. Her charisma mobilized the community health nursing students to engage in fundraising for the memorial as a class project.

2. Have students analyze a policy on a health issue affecting the local community. Find out who benefits and who loses as a result of the policy. Use the policy anlaysis model in Figure 13-2. Follow up on views by writing a letter to a political leader in regard to the policy analyzed.

CLINICAL LABORATORY TEACHING STRATEGIES

1. Have students attend a city council or board of supervisors meeting in their local community. In a clinical conference, share the community health–related policies under discussion at the meeting and determine how the policies came about and whether they need to be changed.

2. Have the students complete a community survey. They should determine the gaps in health service that are of concern to the community, find out who the most active people are in this area of concern, and learn what is being done to alleviate the problem(s). Are the gaps being discussed in city council or board of supervisors' meetings? Who

will bring them to the attention of local politicians? Is this something a group of nursing students could do along with several concerned citizens?

ACTIVITIES TO PROMOTE CRITICAL THINKING IN THE CLASSROOM

1. Investigate major health policy systems in your community or state. Are community health nurses represented in one of the systems? If so, invite her or him to be a guest speaker in your class. Suggest that the speaker address boundaries of the system, authority of the system, resources the system uses, how the system invites or accesses input, and what has been the system's recent output. Allow time for questions, and ask how student community health nurses can assist in the functioning of this system.

2. As an alternative learning experience, create an opportunity for a group of students to meet with a legislator on an important public health issue that requires her or his support to pass or to veto. Assist the students in being prepared (see guidelines in Chapter 13) when talking with legislators. Suggest that the students report their experience to peers during class. Ask them what they did right and what would they do differently if they approached a legislator again?

3. Suggest that several students who are covered by a health insurance plan share specific aspects of the plan with the class. Put a graph on the board that has columns for cost, coverage, co-payments, and so on. With four or five plans represented, discuss the differences in the plans.

4. As part of the course, have small groups of students attend a variety of health planning or health policy meetings (public or private health care agencies, local government agency, etc.). After all have attended at least one meeting, discuss the following questions: How often were finances discussed? Who controlled the discussion? Were meaningful decisions made? Was another meeting called on the same subject or a subcommittee formed to address this subject?

5. During the term have students interact with health care administrators in a variety of agencies and venues and ask the leaders what their views are on health care reform, whether they are in a position to be involved in influencing policy, and whether they are politically active (as leaders in agencies used for clinical laboratory experiences, as guest speakers, as people the students interview, etc.)? Near the end of the term ask the students to share the answers to the three questions.

6. Create a combined list of website addresses for government agencies and organizations from students in the class. Make copies and give to each student as a resource.

■ Evaluation Strategies

MULTIPLE-CHOICE QUESTIONS

1. Health policy should:

Reflect a community's values
Health policy should reflect a community's values and should not only be created for certain groups such as the influential or the poor. It needs to come from the people within the community and be for all of them.

Be made for a few influential people
This is what is to be avoided. Health policy should reflect the needs and values of the community.

Be created by people outside of the community
This is not ideal. The health policy should have a lot of community involvement. Some communities may need the help of experts as they organize their efforts and move along the process, but the creation of the planned policy change should come from within the local community.

Reflect the needs of the community's poor
Depending on the health policy change, all community members' needs must be considered—none at the expense of others and ideally none more than others. There are times when one particular group may be affected more directly, but all community members should benefit.

2. An example of a regulatory health policy includes:

Licensure of health professionals
Regulatory health policy regulates or licenses services or people providing services in the community. Distributive health policy subsidizes nursing education, benefits the needy, and allocates resources among and between groups.

Federal subsidies for nursing education
This is an example of a distributive health policy and is not regulatory.

Benefits for needy groups
This is an example of a distributive health policy and is not regulatory.

Allocating resources among groups
This is an example of a distributive health policy and is not regulatory.

3. The most troubling issue in health care that outweighs all others is:

Cost

In the United States a greater percentage of income is spent on health care than in any other country, and the amount keeps increasing. Other issues, such as accessibility, quality, and special groups of uninsured and underinsured, are significant, but cost remains the most troubling issue.

Physical accessibility

Accessibility in general is a significant concern and must be remedied, but cost is the most troubling issue making health care financially inaccessible to many.

Quality of care

Quality of care is of concern to all people and must be constantly monitored and improved, but cost is the most troubling issue for Americans.

The uninsured

The majority of people (85%) in the United States have some form of insurance (Medicare, Medicaid, private policies, and special programs for children). Although many people still have major gaps in their health insurance coverage, there are more people who find those additional costs prohibitive than the number who are totally uninsured.

4. The legislative process is:

Similar at the state and federal levels

The legislative process is long and detailed, is initiated at the local level, and requires skill, power, money, and patience to pursue it. The processes are similar at the state and federal levels.

A simple process designed for anyone to follow

The legislative process is long and detailed and can be confusing to the uninitiated.

A process that takes about 3 months

The legislative process is long and detailed and can take years. It would be very unusual for a bill to become state or federal law in 3 months.

Not a process in which community health nurses should become involved

It is a process in which nurses should be involved. However, more community health nurses should become involved as they have influence they are not using.

5. Why is it important for community health nurses to understand the legislative process?

The nurse's change agent role includes involvement in the community's political arena.

The political activist role should not be added to a nurse's role description, nor do nurses have the time to become watchdogs to legislators. No one should be in control of health policy at any level. The nurse as a change agent, however, needs to be involved and influential in the community's political arena.

The nurse may decide to add the role of political activist to the nursing role description.

This would be inappropriate to add to a nurse's job description. However, many nurses have strong feelings about a variety of political issues, and nurses should be encouraged to pursue them inside and out of the nursing role.

Nurses need to become watchdogs of the activities of state and federal legislators.

This is a very time-consuming role, and individuals are hired just to do this job. It would be beyond the expectations of a community health nurse.

Legislative knowledge allows the nurse to be in control of health policy in the state.

Legislative knowledge is important, but knowledge alone does not allow the nurse to be in control of the state's health policy. No one person is in control of health policy at the state and federal levels; there are many players in the political arena at these levels.

ESSAY QUESTIONS

1. When you consider the concept of health care reform, what changes do you envision and how will those changes be paid for? What are some of the current health care issues that may be part of smaller health care changes, such as Medicare covering medications for elders or individuals being able to invest a percentage of Social Security in the stock market?

2. Think of your political involvement thus far in your life (working for political candidates, writing letters to legislators, membership in a student nurse organization, etc.). How will that history affect your political involvement when you are a registered nurse?

INDIVIDUAL OR GROUP PROJECTS

1. Select an issue currently before your local, state, or federal legislature and follow the progress of this issue (bill) throughout the semester. At the end of the semester, report to the class on the status of the bill. You may want to involve the class by having

class members write letters to legislators in support of or against the bill.

2. Attend all local meetings or hearings on an issue of concern to you and your community. Present testimony from your perspective as a student in community health nursing and follow the steps outlined in this chapter for generating support when becoming politically involved.

UNIT III

Public Health Principles in Community Health Nursing

CHAPTER 14

Epidemiology in Community Health Care

LEARNING OBJECTIVES

Upon mastery of this chapter, you should be able to:

- Explore the historical roots of epidemiology.

- Explain the host, agent, and environment model.

- Describe theories of causality in health and illness.

- Define immunity and compare passive, active, cross, and herd immunity.

- Explain how epidemiologists determine populations at risk.

- Identify the four stages of a disease or health condition.

- List the major sources of epidemiologic information.

- Distinguish between incidence and prevalence in health and illness states.

- Use epidemiologic methods to describe an aggregate's health.

- Distinguish between types of epidemiologic studies useful for researching aggregate health.

- Use the seven-step research process when conducting an epidemiologic study.

KEY TERMS

Agent	Host
Analytic epidemiology	Immunity
Case-control studies	Incidence
Causality	Morbidity rate
Cohort	Mortality rate
Cross-sectional studies	Natural history
Descriptive epidemiology	Pandemic
Endemic	Prevalence
Environment	Prospective study
Epidemic	Rates
Epidemiology	Retrospective study
Experimental epidemiology	Risk
Experimental study	

■ Teaching Strategies

CLASSROOM TEACHING STRATEGIES

1. Select a topic or have the class identify a problem or concern that is a threat to the health and well-being of their community, such as drug abuse, teenage pregnancies, high school dropout rates, tuberculosis, or sexually transmitted diseases. Guide the class through the seven steps of the epidemiologic investigative process. Demonstrate how the multiple causation theory can be used as a conceptual model for the study developed by the class.

2. Invite a nurse-epidemiologist from a local public health agency to speak to the class about her or his role.

CLINICAL LABORATORY TEACHING STRATEGIES

1. Assign to students clients who need epidemiologic follow-up (such as tuberculosis and *Salmonella* investigations) and have them share their experiences with the other students during a clinical laboratory conference.

2. Encourage students to participate (or observe and ask questions) in epidemiologic studies being conducted by community agencies as part of their clinical laboratory experience. Share the experiences during a clinical laboratory conference.

ACTIVITIES TO PROMOTE CRITICAL THINKING IN THE CLASSROOM

1. Use the class-selected topics arising in teaching strategy 1 (above) and have the class identify the host, agent, and environment factors for each disease or condition.

2. Complete this activity as a class. Select a new topic such as a healthy pregnancy. Schematically diagram the healthy pregnancy to show the web of causation for a healthy state (see pages 254–255 in the textbook).

3. Describe the natural history of a healthy pregnancy, outlining its four stages (see pages 256–257 in the textbook). Identify three preventive nursing interventions used at the primary level of prevention.

4. Using the six questions in critical thinking activity 4 for this chapter, select a study conducted at your university, a graduate student's thesis, or a study you have conducted as an additional example to examine.

5. Ask the nurse-epidemiologist you invited as a speaker (teaching strategy 2 above) to discuss an epidemiologic study recently conducted or currently being conducted at her or his agency. Ask the speaker to describe the study design and outcome.

6. Suggest that the students explore various agencies in their community that serve young mothers and/or high-risk infants. Have them inquire whether the agencies are aware of or use David Olds' model in their work with young families. If they do, share their work with the class. If they do not, share a copy of a recent article outlining his group's work.

▪ Evaluation Strategies

MULTIPLE-CHOICE QUESTIONS

1. The tripartite epidemiologic model includes:

   Host, agent, and environment
   The purpose of this model is to demonstrate the relationship among these three components. Each component has to be present to a certain degree in order for any disease, illness, or injury to exist or happen. If one component is missing, illness or injury will not occur.

   Incidence, prevalence, and case fatality
   Two of these terms describe ways of identifying cases of disease, and case fatality is a term used to determine the number of deaths from a specific disease. They are not terms used in the epidemioligic model.

   Health, illness, and injury
   These terms describe outcomes. They are what occurs when the host, agent, and environment are present in the right proportions.

   Immunity, causation, and risk
   These are additional terms used in epidemiology. They do not refer to the epidemiologic triad.

2. The science of epidemiology is important for community health nurses to understand because:

   Much of their work focuses on the cause and effect of health and illness.
   Community health nurses work with a variety of client and client groups and are expected to base all of their work on the cause and effect of variables that influence health and illness.

   Communicable diseases are rampant in the community.
   This may be true, but epidemiology is a broad science and refers to wellness, non-communicable diseases, and injury as well as communicable diseases.

   They have the ability to prevent mass epidemics.
   This is possible, but it is not the only reason community health nurses should be knowledgeable about epidemiology. Epidemiology is a broad science and refers to wellness, non-communicable diseases, and injury as well as communicable diseases.

   Epidemiology is a new science and nurses should stay current.
   It is an old science with its roots in earliest recorded history and the formal development of epidemiology as a science occurring in the mid-1800s. Nurses should stay current in all aspects of the sciences impacting nursing.

3. Today the epidemiology of wellness is focused on through the use of holistic models of health. Basic to these models is:

   Lifestyle with its self-created risks
   Today there is an increased focus on lifestyle behaviors and how they relate to a person's state of wellness or illness. It is a basic component of a wellness model.

   Communicable disease control
   Communicable disease control focuses on an illness state, not a wellness state, and is not part of a wellness model.

   The natural history of disease
   The four stages of the natural history of a disease or health condition are useful in determining the natural progression of an illness state. It is not part of a wellness model.

   Vital statistics and reportable diseases
   These are sources of record keeping that provide information for epidemiologic study. They are not a part of a wellness model.

4. A cross-control study is an observational study that:

   Compares persons with a health-illness condition and persons without the condition
   Comparing persons with and without a certain condition is known as a case-control study.

   Describes patterns of occurrence of illness and injury in a population
   This describes a descriptive study, which observes and describes the patterns of illness and injury occurrence in populations.

   Investigates the development of health-illness conditions over a long period of time
   This describes a longitudinal study. There are many famous studies where populations have been followed over decades, always providing new information, such as the Framingham Heart Study and the Harvard Women's Health Study.

   Studies a cohort and evaluates variables associated with the disease or injury
   This describes a cohort study. In a cohort study one group of people, such as WWI veterans, Holocaust survivors, or year 2000 high school graduates, are studied over time.

5. A community trial is:

   A type of experimental study conducted at the community level
   A community trial is conducted as an experimental study design with large populations. Some of the community receives a treatment, while the other part does not. The Kingston/Newberg study using fluoridated water is a classic community trial.

   An inexpensive type of analytic study
   This is probably the most expensive type of experimental study. It involves a great number of subjects, the support of the governmental forces as well as the population involved, a large number of staff over a long period of time, and the cost of the intervention itself.

   A study that gathers volunteers for the experimental group
   When a whole community is involved, individuals are not approached to be volunteers. What makes it a community study is that the entire community is part of the study.

   A way to locate health problems in a variety of communities
   The health problem is identified prior to the implementation of the study. The introduction of an intervention in one community with no introduction in a similar community forms the study population, and the health problem being studied is then monitored between the two populations. The health problem has to be identified first in this type of study.

6. The concept of causality refers to:

   The relationship between a cause and its effect
   The concept of causality looks for the connections between cause and effect. There is a chain of causality, and at times causes may be multiple and complex.

   All the possible influences on the health and illness processes
   This describes a very broad view of causation. It is broader than one web of causation, which looks at all the possible influences on illness, and a second web of causation developed to determine all influences on wellness.

   The host's ability to resist infectious disease–causing agents
   This describes immunity, which can be natural (such as related to race, ethnicity, or sex) or acquired (such as through immunization).

   The chances that a disease or health problem will occur
   This pertains to the risk or the probability that a disease or other unfavorable health condition will develop.

ESSAY QUESTIONS

1. Using the seven steps of the epidemiologic process, follow a specific community health illness or injury condition through the steps. Identify how a study on the selected topic could be conducted locally with the resources known to be available.

2. Identify a community health issue of importance to you. What studies do you feel need to be conducted on this topic? How could you go about beginning to research this issue? What agencies might you involve or go to for more information on this problem at the local level?

INDIVIDUAL OR GROUP PROJECTS

1. Assign student(s) to visit the local health department office of statistics or research to observe how data are obtained, recorded, and analyzed. Have the student(s) report observations to the clinical laboratory group or classmates.

2. Using a research article that includes an epidemiologic study, have students design a similar investigation in their own community. Needed modifications and changes in the design should be included. This is intended to be a paper-and-pencil exercise but may develop into an actual study if the opportunity presents itself.

CHAPTER 15

Communicable Disease Control

LEARNING OBJECTIVES

Upon mastery of this chapter, you should be able to:

- Discuss the global and national trends and issues in communicable disease control.

- Describe the three modes of transmission for communicable diseases.

- Explain the strategies used for the three levels of prevention in communicable disease control.

- Explain the significance of immunization as a communicable disease control measure.

- Describe major issues impacting the control and elimination of tuberculosis.

- Differentiate between HIV infection and AIDS.

- Discuss specific ways to prevent sexually transmitted diseases, including HIV/AIDS.

- Identify six globally emerging communicable diseases.

- Describe the nurse's role in communicable disease control.

- Discuss ethical issues affecting communicable disease and infection control.

KEY TERMS

Acquired immunodeficiency
  syndrome (AIDS)
Active immunity
Communicable disease
Direct transmission
Fomites
Herd immunity
Human immunodeficiency
  (HIV)
Immunization
Incubation period

Indirect transmission
Infectious
Isolation
Passive immunity
Quarantine
Reservoir
Screening
Surveillance
Vaccine
Vector

■Teaching Strategies

CLASSROOM TEACHING STRATEGIES

1. Invite an epidemiologist-clinician from an STD clinic to discuss local trends in STD incidence and control. Perhaps the speaker has slides of classic and common STDs to enhance the presentation.

2. Invite the leader of an AIDS support group or a family and friends of AIDS clients' support group to talk to the class. Ask the speaker to focus on the role of the nurse that she or he feels is most important when working with AIDS clients.

CLINICAL LABORATORY TEACHING STRATEGIES

1. Encourage students to spend clinical laboratory time in an STD clinic in a participatory or observer role. The main objective should be to explore the care provider's role, caregiving technique, and counseling style. The student should write a critique of this experience.

2. Allow students to participate in an immunization clinic. Provide an inservice on immunization administration (if needed or as review) and have students participate in well-baby immunization clinics, flu clinics for older adults (fall or winter term), or as part of a TB skin-testing program. Discuss the collective experiences among all students near the end of the clinical laboratory experience.

ACTIVITIES TO PROMOTE CRITICAL THINKING IN THE CLASSROOM

1. If possible, invite a state health department epidemiologist or local health department epidemiologist to talk to the class. Have her or him share how communicable disease surveillance is conducted and which communicable diseases are posing the greatest threat to the health of citizens in your state and/or local community.

2. Use a recent issue of *Mortality and Morbidity Weekly Report* and compare communicable disease issues discussed with those found in a copy of the same publication from 10, 15, or 20 years ago. What has changed and what is the same?

3. Discuss the local rates of immunization among preschool children in your city or county. Is it at a safe herd immunity level (see page 300 in the textbook)? Suggest that the students propose some recommendations for preserving or raising this level.

4. Repeat the activity in class by discussing several high-risk populations discussed in this chapter and determining what factors make these groups vulnerable to specific communicable diseases. Are there additional published sources that provide support for the class's opinions? Suggest that the students propose at least one nursing intervention appropriate for a group and outline how it might be accomplished.

5. Provide an opportunity for some of the students to complete a contact investigation form on a client or clients in the clinical laboratory experience (on a shared visit with a staff public health nurse or alone). This may be a usual activity for all students. In either case, allow the students to share the following: How did they preserved privacy and confidentiality? What measures have proved most effective in reaching contacts? What is the students' evaluation of the success?

6. Suggest that the students access the CDC through the Internet (http://www.cdc.gov) and have them click on hoaxes and rumors. You might want to have the students do this every 2 to 3 weeks and hold a discussion near the end of the term. What misinformation is currently being circulated about how diseases are contracted and what diseases are being transmitted? How different is this information from what clients might believe? In fact, have the students ask their clients on home visit how they believe specific diseases (gonorrhea, syphilis, AIDS, etc.) are transmitted. The students might find that lay beliefs, national hoaxes, and rumors are very similar.

■ Evaluation Strategies

MULTIPLE-CHOICE QUESTIONS

1. As a nation we have experienced a dramatic decrease in this disease since 1990. In fact, there were 278 cases per 100,000 in that year, and in 1997 there were 122 per 100,000, exceeding the *Healthy People 2000* goals. The goal for 2010 for this disease is 19 per 100,000. This disease is:

Gonorrhea
We have seen dramatic reductions in gonorrhea in the past decade, and these figures accurately represent those significant changes.

Syphilis
The incidence of this disease had decreased in recent years, but the numbers of cases has been smaller than for gonorrhea. In 1997 we exceeded the Healthy People 2000 *goal of 4 per 100,000, and the 2010 goal is 0.25 per 100,000.*

Chlamydia
The incidence of this disease remains high, with 4 million acute infections each year. The Healthy People 2010 *goal for chlamydia in 15- to 24-year-olds is 300 per 100,000.*

Viral warts
Twenty million Americans carry the virus, and 1 million new cases are diagnosed each year. It remains a major communicable disease.

2. HIV/AIDS presents an intriguing and complex service delivery problem due to issues such as:

Sexual behaviors, illegal drug use and end-of-life issues
There are many factors that interplay in the AIDS epidemic; however, sexual behavior, illegal drug use, and end-of-life issues are three major ones. The multidimensional services, caregiver attitudes, and perhaps legal violations of drug abuse that surround AIDS clients complicate caregiving.

The highly vulnerable and risky position in which it places caregivers
All people in caregiving positions with anyone should use universal precautions. They should be the norm and not the exception. When universal precautions are used, caregivers are not vulnerable or at risk.

The negative attitude HIV/AIDS clients have toward caregivers
There is no evidence that HIV/AIDS clients have negative attitudes toward caregivers.

Which of the curative treatments are best to use
*Unfortunately, at this time there is no cure for
HIV/AIDS. However, there are life-extending
combinations of medications for the HIV-
positive client.*

3. There are three major goals to be achieved with the
HIV-infected population. Which of the following is
one of them?

Delaying the onset of clinical symptoms with
antiviral therapy
*The three goals are: (1) promoting general health
and resilience, (2) preventing infections of all
sorts, and (3) delaying the onset of clinical
symptoms with antiviral therapy.*

Achieving a speedy and comfortable death
*Life without an AIDS diagnosis for the HIV client
can be prolonged for years with combination
drug therapy. If AIDS develops, the focus should
still be on a quality life. If death is inevitable it
should be a comfortable one, not necessarily a
speedy one.*

Decreasing the intensity of infections the HIV client
acquires
*A goal is to prevent infections of all sorts and not
the intensity of infections. Of course, if an
infection occurs prompt treatment will decrease
the intensity.*

Locating housing options as the AIDS client's health
deteriorates
*This may be an item within a nursing care plan but
is not one of the major goals of care, as not all
AIDS clients will need such an option.*

4. Tuberculosis Classification III means the person
has:

A positive skin test and positive chest x-ray
*Classification III is the classification for TB disease.
Clients have had exposure, a positive skin test,
and positive chest x-ray and/or sputum tests.*

What is called a TB infection
*A history of exposure and a positive skin test is
Classification II or TB infection.*

A less severe case of TB than those with
Classification V
*Classification V is reserved for a TB suspect with
evaluation not completed.*

Less of a chance of getting TB than if he or she had
Classification I and II
*Classification III is TB disease. This person has
gone through Classification 0 (no exposure), I
(exposure), and II (exposure and a positive skin
test and a negative chest x-ray).*

5. Tuberculosis Classification I means the person has:

A history of being exposed to TB
*Classification I means the person has been exposed
to TB. Some persons do not know that they have
been exposed; others know.*

A positive skin test and positive chest x-ray
*Classification III is the classification for TB disease.
Clients have had exposure, a positive skin test,
and positive chest x-ray and/or sputum tests.*

What is called a TB infection
*A history of exposure and a positive skin test is
Classification II or TB infection.*

A less severe case of TB than those with
Classification V
*Classification V is reserved for a TB suspect with
evaluation not completed.*

6. Which of the following is an example of primary
prevention and communicable disease control?

Administering immunizations to senior citizens at a
flu clinic
*This is an example of primary prevention—
preventing the disease from occurring.*

Administering TB skin test to children entering
kindergarten
*This is an example of secondary prevention—
prompt diagnosis and treatment.*

Providing chest x-rays to people with positive TB
skin tests
*This is an example of secondary prevention—
prompt diagnosis and treatment.*

Receiving prompt treatment for the symptoms of
gonorrhea
*This is an example of secondary prevention—
prompt diagnosis and treatment.*

7. Hepatitis B is a global viral infection transmitted by
the following method:

Exposure to contaminated blood or serous fluids
*This can occur in certain high-risk groups, including
injected drug users, heterosexuals with multiple
partners, and homosexual men. It can also occur
when occupationally exposed to contaminated
blood or serous fluids.*

The oral–fecal route of transmission
This is the method of transmission for Hepatitis A.

Air-borne droplet nuclei
*This air-borne method of disease transmission is
related to TB and is not how Hepatitis B is
transmitted.*

Infected rodents, such as mice and rats
This is not the method of transmitting Hepatitis B.

ESSAY QUESTIONS

1. Express your thoughts in approximately 200 words by using the following introductory sentence that you will complete: "If I cared for an AIDS client in her or his home I would feel..."

2. In the United States the TB skin test (Mantoux, PPD) is used as the standard method for evaluating TB infection. In other countries the BCG vaccine is used routinely. Explain how you feel about each choice and give your rationale.

INDIVIDUAL OR GROUP PROJECTS

1. Assist in a survey of the entire population of a senior citizen housing unit receiving flu and pneumonia immunizations, either from a personal health care provider or a flu clinic. Inquire into reasons why some people did not receive the vaccines. Are all medically eligible seniors receiving the vaccines? Why or why not? What can a community health nurse do about it?

2. Spend time with a school nurse as children entering kindergarten are assessed for immunization compliance. What barriers existed for families of underimmunized or unimmunized children? What percent were underimmunized or unimmunized? Discuss these issues with the school nurse and ask how she or he resolves the problems.

CHAPTER 16

Environmental Health and Safety

LEARNING OBJECTIVES

Upon mastery of this chapter, you should be able to:

- Discuss the importance of applying an ecologic perspective to any investigation of human–environment relationships.

- Explain the concepts of prevention and long-range environmental impact and their importance for environmental health.

- Discuss at least five global environmental concerns, and describe hazards associated with each area.

- Relate the effect of the above hazards on people's health.

- Discuss appropriate interventions for addressing the above environmental health problems, including community health nursing's role.

- Describe how national health objectives for the year 2010 target environmental health.

- Describe strategies for nursing collaboration and participation in efforts to promote and protect environmental health.

KEY TERMS

Contaminant	Environmental impact
Deforestation	Environmental justice
Demographic entrapment	Extinction
Desertification	Global warming
Ecologic perspective	Pollution
Ecosystem	Toxic agent
Environmental health	Wetlands

■Teaching Strategies

CLASSROOM TEACHING STRATEGIES

1. Invite an environmental engineer, a representative of the Environmental Protection Agency (EPA) or the Occupational Safety and Health Administration (OSHA), or other appropriate speakers from the local health department to speak to the class about environmental hazards in the community and what is being done about them.

2. Assign the students to develop a home environmental hazards checklist, and suggest that they use it with clients they visit in their clinical laboratory experience.

CLINICAL LABORATORY TEACHING STRATEGIES

1. Have the students conduct a windshield survey (see Chapter 18) of a selected geographic area to identify environmental hazards. Assign the students to diverse geographical areas (industrial, residential, commercial, rural, and high-density urban) to make comparisons of the kinds of hazards present.

2. During home visits to assigned client families, ask the students to assess home environments for obvious health hazards, using the checklist that was developed as a class assignment.

ACTIVITIES TO PROMOTE CRITICAL THINKING IN THE CLASSROOM

1. Develop a hypothetical family and environment they live in that will include several environmental hazards. Have students use the nursing process to develop a plan to improve the environment. Place the scenario on a screen in front of the room so each student can read it, or hand out copies of the scenario. Suggest that the students trade papers in some organized fashion and critique one another's plans. Collectively develop one plan that takes the best suggestions from the class to use as a model for everyone.

2. Discuss some of the potential environmental hazards students have been observing in their clinical laboratory settings. For example, are there people living near polluted creeks, families living near large factories, or an elementary school built under or next to high-tension wires? Develop an approach that would satisfactorily prevent populations from being at risk from the examples the students share in class. What agencies might be needed to assist? What can the community health nurse do?

3. Have the students peruse the local newspaper(s) for a few weeks looking for stories about environmental health problems, such as the Firestone tire problem of 2000 or a more local issue occurring in your community. Ask questions in activity 3 (page 335) for student feedback.

4. Show the environmental checklist designed in the classroom teaching strategy 2 (above) to one of the speakers from the EPA or OSHA (teaching strategy 1 above), and ask him or her to review it before using it in the clinical laboratory setting.

5. Select one environmental health issue occurring locally, and with the students this term pursue it to be as informed about the problem as possible. Use all the steps identified in activity 5. By taking the students through this process, they will have first-hand experience for future issues they may want or need to pursue when they are employed as nurses.

6. Suggest that if the students conduct group teaching projects, at least one should be on the topic of environmental safety. Modify this group-teaching plan to be used by all students with families on home visits.

7. Discuss what steps a community health nurse could engage in to promote the development of policies and legislation that would enhance consumer protection and promote a healthier environment.

8. Select a program that is in place to improve an environmental health issue, such as cleaning up an oil spill and saving affected wildlife or another current issue. Discuss how you would determine the effectiveness of the program. What should be in the evaluation plan for the program?

9. Discuss some environmentally related research that is being conducted at your university. Were/are any of the students involved in the research? Is there a possibility of any students participating in any currently planned environmentally related university research? Explore these possibilities in conjunction with faculty who teach at the graduate level and who might have master's students doing environmental research.

■ Evaluation Strategies

MULTIPLE-CHOICE QUESTIONS

1. An ecological perspective of environmental health is:

   The recognition that we affect the environment and the environment affects us
   The total relationship or patterns of relationships between people and their environment is known as the ecological perspective.

   The study of governmental and private sector regulations of the environment
   Such a study does not define the scope of an ecological perspective of environmental health.

   A technological view of strategies for preventing illness and injury
   Such a view does not define the scope of an ecological perspective of environmental health.

   The role of the community health nurse in preventing injury, disease, and illness
   The nurse's role includes the three levels of the prevention of environmental health and safety issues and is aware of the ecological perspective.

2. A vector is defined as:

   Non-human carriers of disease organisms that can transmit disease directly to humans
   A vector is a non-human carrier of disease organisms that can transmit these organisms directly to humans.

   A chemical, either natural or synthetic, that is capable of acting as a carcinogen
   A chemical is the agent that causes a disease and is not referred to as a vector. A vector is a living, non-human carrier and not the agent.

   An infectious agent carried to humans through food sources
   A vector is the carrier of the infectious agent and not the agent itself.

   Toxic substances introduced by humans into the underground water supply
   A vector is the carrier of the infectious or toxic agent and not the agent itself.

3. The issue of water pollution is:

   Significant because it causes millions of episodes of disease in the country each year
   Water pollution is not new and is a problem in all water sources in the United States, as well as other countries. It causes millions of cases of diseases yearly, some mild and some severe enough to cause death.

A new one due to the proliferation of industries in the United States
Water pollution is not a new problem; in fact, it is an old problem that escalated during the Industrial Revolution and has continued in all countries.

A major problem in other countries, but not in the United States
Water pollution is a major problem in all countries. Some countries, including the United States, have the resources to identify the problem and do something about it.

Nonexistent in ground water sources, the use of which should be increased
Pollution has leached into ground water, especially from agricultural pesticides.

4. The EPA was established in 1971, mainly to:

Give authority over environmental issues that affect the public's health
The EPA was established to have authority over all environmental matters regarding the protection of the public's health.

Identify and address world health issues
This is the role of the World Health Organization (WHO).

Protect occupational safety and health
This is the role of the Occupational Safety and Health Administration (OSHA).

Monitor food and drug production and availability
This is the role of the Food and Drug Administration (FDA).

5. Deforestation and desertification are environmental health concerns. These are identified by:

Clearing land and converting it into wasteland
Unchecked logging and land clearing operations in forests and in the tropics cause deforestation. Denuding fertile lands by diverting water supplies causes desertification. Both are effected by political decisions and have a major negative impact on global health.

Unhealthy or contaminated food
This is identified by foods made unhealthy due to pollution or contamination by toxic substances and is a separate issue from deforestation and desertification.

Insect and rodent control
This is identified by methods employed to decrease vectors that can carry disease and is a separate issue from deforestation and desertification.

Energy depletion
This is identified by depletion of major energy sources, especially from fossil fuels, before alternative methods are developed and widely used. Deforestation and desertification is a separate issue.

6. Radon exposure is of increasing concern. Radon exposure occurs by:

Inhaling the solid, radioactive decay products of radon gas seeping through the ground into homes from the soil
This describes how radon exposure occurs.

Toddlers and preschoolers ingesting peeling paint from older homes or playing in contaminated soil
This describes how lead poisoning can occur.

Exposing oneself to the sun's rays without sun-screening lotions or protective clothing
This describes exposure to radiation from the sun, which can have untoward long-term effects.

Inhaling the odorless and colorless gas produced by engine combustion, which can cause death
This describes exposure to and possible outcomes from carbon monoxide gas inhalation.

7. Sunbathing is:

Not recommended regardless of skin tone, age, altitude, or part of the world
This is true. Sun exposure should be minimized and SPF 30-lotion or protective clothing should be worn even for short periods of time outdoors.

Safe if done for short periods of time on cloudy days
Sunbathing is not a safe practice, and you burn even on cloudy days.

Recommended if a sun-screening lotion with SPF 60 or higher is used
Sunbathing is never recommended, but if outdoors, a lotion with SPF 30 should be used, which is the highest level made.

Only for children because as you age your skin is more sensitive and it is unsafe
Children's skin is very sensitive, and they should be protected whenever outdoors. Exposure to the sun is cumulative, and exposure as a child can cause health problems years later.

ESSAY QUESTIONS

1. Think about a population of senior citizens. Select two living arrangements common to elders and identify possible environmental hazards that may impact their health and well-being. Are there major differences between the two living arrangements selected?

2. Select an article researching an environmental health issue in a copy of the *American Journal of Public Health*. Copy the abstract and distribute it to the class members. Ask the students to write a reaction to the problem in the study and determine how the study could be replicated in your community.

INDIVIDUAL OR GROUP PROJECTS

1. Mentally, go through your home and list each room and your yard. Identify all potential environmental health hazards. Identify how you would make the needed changes.

2. Divide the class into 5 or 10 groups. Each group should select one (or two) of the 10 categories of environmental concerns and research it locally. Explore your city or county for strengths and weaknesses in each area. Verbally report the findings to the class.

3. Ask students to bring newspaper articles to class that report on local, regional, or state environmental health issues and share them throughout the duration of the course. Allow a few minutes during several classes to discuss each article. This could be voluntary or part of a class participation grade.

UNIT IV

Community as Client

CHAPTER 17

Theoretical Basis of Community Health Nursing

LEARNING OBJECTIVES

Upon mastery of this chapter, you should be able to:

- Discuss two essential characteristics of nursing service when a community is the client: community-oriented, population-focused care, and relationship-based care.

- Describe the contributions of at least six models of nursing practice to community health.

- Explain the benefits of applying eight tenets of public health nursing to community health nursing.

- Identify at least five social issues that influence contemporary community health nursing care.

KEY TERMS

Bioterrorism	Model
Community-oriented, population-focused care	Relationship-based care
	Technology
Genetic engineering	Tenet
Global economy	Theory
Migration	

■ Teaching Strategies

CLASSROOM TEACHING STRATEGIES

1. Take the main concepts from pages 341 to 342 in the textbook and facilitate a class discussion on the terms community-oriented, population-focused care and relationship-based care. Discover what these terms mean to the students, especially now that they have been in the clinical laboratory settings for awhile.

2. Ask the students to choose one of the six nursing practice models presented in this chapter and use it to describe clients they have worked with thus far in the clinical laboratory.

CLINICAL LABORATORY TEACHING STRATEGIES

1. Among the selected activities you expect students to become involved in during clinical laboratory time, select at least one population-focused activity. This can be an immunization clinic, teaching groups of pregnant teens or elders, or any other opportunity the setting offers.

2. During a clinical conference, discuss the eight tenets of public health and ask students to describe instances where these tenets were incorporated into their clinical laboratory activities.

ACTIVITIES TO PROMOTE CRITICAL THINKING IN THE CLASSROOM

1. After the students have been in the clinical laboratory setting for 4 to 6 weeks, ask them the following three questions: What population-focused services does the agency provide? How might the community health nurse expand the present population-based services? What is the nurse's role in the assessment, development, implementation, and evaluation of these programs?

2. Since teaching is a major role of the community health nurse, use any opportunity to ask students (either in class or in the clinical laboratory setting) to verbalize how an educational intervention would be used with the client group being discussed. This simple exercise helps to keep students thinking in terms of educating populations to create a population more involved in its own care.

3. Whenever discussing the health care needs of an individual client or a family client, have the students expand their thought processes by discussing what additional factors should be considered for assessment and intervention that would indicate an aggregate or community-focused approach.

4. In this chapter, five societal issues are described. In addition, six nursing practice models are discussed. Choose one nursing practice model and determine how it would guide a nurse's approach to managing, improving, or possibly eliminating the negative aspects of the societal issue. Repeat the exercise with additional models from the textbook or the model used by your school or clinical laboratory agency.

5. Suggest that the students select one of the societal influences on the community or populations and find the latest information on that subject on the Internet. Determine a particular class to which they are to bring their information to share and discuss.

■Evaluation Strategies

MULTIPLE-CHOICE QUESTIONS

1. A nursing practice model that focuses on self-care is the model proposed by:

Orem
She is the nursing theorist who proposed this model whereby nurses function to meet clients' self-care needs until they are able to do so for themselves.

Nightingale
She is the nursing theorist who proposed an environmental theory that focuses on preventive care to populations.

Neuman
She is the nursing theorist who proposed a systems model that is adapted in community health nursing to view clients as aggregates.

Rogers
She is the nursing theorist who developed a systems model emphasizing the whole client and incorporating the development of "unity" persons.

2. A community health nurse using Roy's nursing practice model when working with a community that is dealing with a particular health issue is involved in:

Assessing a community's coping mechanisms to have the community use its collective abilities to promote adaptation
This is the premise of Roy's Adaptation Model and a description of how the community health nurse would be guided by her model.

Assessing a community's lines of resistance and defense to stresses in the internal and external environment
This is the premise of Neuman's Health Care Systems Model applied in the community.

Assessing a community for environmental conditions and working to improve negative conditions
This is the premise of Nightingale's Environmental Theory. The crux of her theory is that poor environmental conditions are bad for health and that good environmental conditions reduce disease.

Assessing a community for its collective ability for independence and self-care
This is the premise of Orem's Self-Care Model; when a community is unable to meet its self-care needs, community health nursing interventions assist until the community is able to provide its own self-care.

3. When a community health nurse applies the public health tenet of targeting all who might benefit from her or his practice, an example of this includes:

Examining policies or programs to determine whether they are accessible and acceptable to a population in need
This is an example of tenet 5—ensuring that those who might benefit are being targeted.

Ensuring that people live in conditions conductive to health
This is an example of tenet 4—promoting a healthful environment.

Promoting a higher level of wellness and preventing health problems
This is an example of tenet 3—focusing on primary prevention.

Ensuring that the community is using limited resources in a way that leads to the greatest improvement in health
This is an example of tenet 7—promoting optimum allocation of resources.

4. In this chapter several major societal issues are mentioned and what community health nurses can do is discussed. Which of the following dramatizes the nurse's role regarding bioterrorism?

A community health nurse ensures that adequate surveillance systems are in place for early detection.
This is one of the actions a community health nurse should take concerning bioterrorism.

A community health nurse educates communities so they can make decisions that best fit their value systems.

This is one of the actions a community health nurse should take concerning genetic engineering.

A community health nurse educates the public about the potential dangers of continuing to contaminate the environment.

This is one of the actions a community health nurse should take concerning climate changes.

A community health nurse advocates for policies that will reduce adverse effects of poverty and income disparities.

This is one of the actions a community health nurse should take concerning global economy.

5. It is important to determine the worth of health information found on the Internet. One way to do this is to:

Look at the date of publication and references included

If these are not included, the information source may be weak or slanted and the information may not be credible.

Determine whether you like the information you are gathering

Liking something is nice but is not a valuable component of the worth of information.

Select one of the first three sites listed because they put the best ones first

This is not recommended. You may have to open several sites before you find the information you are looking for, and the order of sites is not a determination of worth.

Avoid ".com" websites because they are promoting their views for financial gains.

Although this means commercial and a product may be involved, this does not automatically affect the quality of the information. In fact, the information may meet all of the factors to determine worth shown in Display 17-3 on page 348.

ESSAY QUESTIONS

1. Select one of the eight tenets of public health and describe how you used it in your work with an assigned family in the clinical laboratory experience.

2. Using the nursing practice model followed in this nursing program (or one from the textbook if the nursing program does not follow a specific model), describe how it guides you when working with a 16-year-old mother of a 6-month-old infant.

INDIVIDUAL OR GROUP PROJECTS

1. Suggest that a group of students assess the need for a population-based service and during the term plan, implement, and evaluate the service that they provided.

2. Suggest that a group of four to six students explore the most recent information on major societal issues impacting public health and create a file of information that is kept in the classroom or clinical laboratory site as a reference during the term. At the end of the term, present the information to the staff members of the clinical laboratory agency for their reference.

CHAPTER 18

The Community as Client: Assessment and Diagnosis

LEARNING OBJECTIVES

Upon mastery of this chapter, you should be able to:

- Describe the meaning of community as client.

- Discuss how a key American value and three myths can undermine a nurses's intention to move beyond an individualistic focus to practice population-based community health nursing.

- Articulate specific considerations of each of the three dimensions of the community as client.

- Express the meaning and significance of community dynamics.

- Compare and contrast five types of community needs assessment.

- Discuss community needs assessment methods.

- Describe four sources of community data.

- Discuss the significance of community diagnoses formation.

- Explain the characteristics of a healthy community.

KEY TERMS

Assets assessment	Individualism
Client myth	Location myth
Community as client	Location variables
Community collaboration	Outcome criteria
Community diagnoses	Population variables
Community needs assessment	Problem-oriented assessment
Community subsystem assessment	Skills myth
Comprehensive assessment	Social system variables
Descriptive epidemiologic study	Survey
Familiarization assessment	Social class

■ Teaching Strategies

CLASSROOM TEACHING STRATEGIES

1. Obtain copies of various individual and family assessment tools used by nurses practicing in a variety of settings. Compare the tools and discuss the merits of each.

2. Designate a locale familiar to all students (such as their own hometown or the university campus) and have students use the three-part Community Profile Inventory (textbook pages 356, 358, and 360) to assess and identify sources of information. Have them use the questions from the profile to develop an assessment of their community from the dimensions of location, population, and social system.

CLINICAL LABORATORY TEACHING STRATEGIES

1. Using the information gathered in classroom teaching strategy 1, design a tool (in conjunction with the clinical laboratory agency administration and staff) to use in the clinical laboratory setting. Pilot the tool, make necessary changes, and suggest the staff use the tool to see whether they find it helpful.

2. Identify the census tracts of the city in which the students have their clinical laboratory experiences. Have groups of students conduct a comprehensive community assessment of each census tract using the three-part Community Profile Inventory on pages 356, 358, and 360 in the textbook. Share the findings during a clinical conference.

ACTIVITIES TO PROMOTE CRITICAL THINKING IN THE CLASSROOM

1. Facilitate a classroom discussion about the importance of understanding and working with the community as a total entity.

2. Facilitate a classroom discussion about viewing the community as client. List specific examples of how this concept is applied in the clinical laboratory experiences of these students.

3. Use the steps in the Activities to Promote Critical Thinking on page 372 in the textbook to explore the health needs of other populations in the community, such as preschoolers, the poor, immigrant groups, or specific religious groups. Are the health needs of such diverse groups different?

4. Discuss when a familiarization or "windshield survey" form of a needs assessment is appropriate. Expect each student to conduct one in his or her clinical laboratory setting. Discuss additional aspects that could be added to this type of assessment, such as stopping and getting out of the car or off of the bus, introducing yourself to shopkeepers in the neighborhood, visiting public buildings and schools, chatting with community officials and teachers, and chatting with key formal and informal leaders as a way of introducing yourself to community members and familiarizing them with your role.

5. Invite someone from the state or local health department who has conducted a community needs assessment survey to speak to the nursing students. Ask him or her to share the process he or she used. Compare the survey process with the suggested steps for conducting a survey described on page 366 in the textbook.

6. Ask students to find surveys available on the Internet or in popular magazines on a variety of subjects. Critique these surveys for the completion of the three phases suggested in the textbook on page 366. How well are these surveys developed?

■ Evaluation Strategies

MULTIPLE-CHOICE QUESTIONS

1. Population-focused practice is best described by which of the following nursing activities?

    Speaking to city council members about the need for additional senior services
    This example depicts a population focus, which is a prime mission of community health nurses.

    Assisting a factory worker injured in an occupational accident
    This example depicts an individual focus. The factory employees are the population focused on, but this demonstrates working with a single employee.

    Checking an elementary school child's hair for signs of lice and nits
    This example depicts an individual focus. The children in the school and the school employees are the population focused on, but this demonstrates working with a single child.

    Counseling a young man about safe sex and the risk of contracting HIV/AIDS
    This example depicts an individual focus. Teaching a group of young men about the same subject would be an example of a population focus.

2. You are part of a health planning team to determine the needs of pregnant teenagers in your community. Which of the following population variables would you want to assess?

    Health needs and practices of subculture groups
    Pregnant teens are a subculture of teenagers. Cultural differences are population variables. Health needs vary among subculture and ethnic populations.

    Location of health services
    The location of health services are location variables.

    Functions of community organizations
    The functions of community organizations are social system variables.

    Level of agreement on community goals
    The level of agreement on community goals are social system variables.

THE FOLLOWING SITUATION APPLIES TO
QUESTIONS 3 THROUGH 5

Nursing students in a community health nursing
course identified toxic waste disposal to be a major
problem in their community.

3. The most cost-effective type of community
assessment to determine the extent of the problem
and the resources available to handle it would be a:

Problem-oriented assessment
*The problem-oriented assessment is commonly used
when familiarization is not sufficient and a
comprehensive assessment is too expensive and
not needed.*

Familiarization assessment
*This type of assessment is not sufficient to
determine the extent of the problem.*

Community subsystem assessment
*A subsystem assessment is too narrow to determine
the extent of the problem.*

Comprehensive community assessment
*This type of community assessment is broader than
needed and is very expensive.*

4. The students conducted a survey to determine
community awareness of the problem of toxic
waste disposal. The final and most important step
in conducting a survey is to:

Report the implications and recommendations of
the survey results
*This is the last and most important step. If the data
are not reported, community awareness and
changes cannot be achieved.*

Develop the survey questionnaire or interview guide
*This occurs during the planning phase in the first
phase of conducting a survey.*

Process data and determine relationships
*This is part of the data analysis, which occurs prior
to the presentation phase.*

Collect data using a valid and reliable tool
*This is not the final step in conducting a survey but
is part of the pretesting and adjusting of the
instrument in the data collection phase or second
phase of conducting a survey.*

5. The data obtained from the community assessment
and survey were used as the basis for developing a
health program. A good way to begin program
implementation would be to:

Ask the city council to hold a town meeting to
discuss the problem
*This demonstrates a population-focused approach
to informing the public and enlisting their help
in solving the toxic waste problem in their
community.*

Plan a cleanup committee made up of student
nurses
*This is unsafe for those participating and will not
solve the continuing problem of toxic waste
existing or being dumped in the community.*

Petition the state government about the danger of
genetic problems
*It may be important to get the state involved in the
problem, and this idea may come from the
people at the town hall meeting. More ideas need
to be generated quickly to solve the problem,
and beginning with the state on genetic problems
is a slow process. Also, has it been determined
that the toxic waste in the community causes
genetic problems?*

Write to a local news station or a national TV news
hour for public disclosure
*It may be important to get the news media involved
in the problem, and this idea may come from the
people at the town hall meeting. Many ideas
need to be generated quickly to solve the
problem, and beginning with a major public
disclosure approach may hinder the process.*

ESSAY QUESTIONS

1. Select one dimension of a community you are
familiar with. Use the community assessment
questions from the three-part Community Profile
Inventory on pages 356, 358, and 360 in the
textbook. Answer the questions in relation to the
community selected.

2. Select one of the five types of community needs
assessment discussed in this chapter. Using either
teenage pregnancy or the aging population, identify
how the community assessment you chose will help
with promoting the health of the population at the
local level.

INDIVIDUAL OR GROUP PROJECTS

1. Using classroom teaching strategy 1 and clinical laboratory teaching strategy 1, modify them to create an individual or group project in class or in the clinical laboratory experience.

2. Select a community you are familiar with. Outline a strategy to assess the community using one of the needs assessment methods discussed in this chapter. Share your rationale for selecting the method chosen before outlining the steps you will take. Develop nursing diagnoses based on assessment data.

CHAPTER 19

Planning, Intervention, and Evaluation of Health Care in Communities

LEARNING OBJECTIVES

Upon mastery of this chapter, you should be able to:

- Describe the nursing process components of planning, implementing, and evaluating as they apply to community health nursing.

- Discuss methods the community health nurse uses to interact with the community.

- Identify the four phases of developing a plan for meeting the health needs in the community.

- Identify actions taken when implementing health promotion activities with aggregates.

- Describe the process of evaluating aggregate health interventions.

- Discuss characteristics of the nursing process affecting nursing practice with the community as client.

- Describe the role of the community health nurse as a catalyst for community development.

KEY TERMS

Coalition	Interaction
Community development	Objectives
Evaluation	Partnerships
Goals	Planning
Implementation	Setting priorities

■ Teaching Strategies

CLASSROOM TEACHING STRATEGIES

1. Ask a community health nurse (public health, school nurse, occupational health nurse) to discuss with the class a community health problem in which the nursing process was utilized to resolve the problem. Ask the nurse to discuss three aspects of the actions taken. Did he or she use a model to assist with the planning phase? Which model and how did it work? What outcomes were he or she looking for? How did he or she conduct the evaluation?

2. Have the students compare and contrast how the nursing process—especially the planning, intervention, and evaluation phases—are used to solve public health problems in a variety of settings where well and ill clients are served.

CLINICAL LABORATORY TEACHING STRATEGIES

1. Ask the students to develop a nursing care plan or plan of action to improve an identified public health problem. This plan should be based on a community assessment (Chapter 18) conducted in the community that the agency serves.

2. Ask the students to discuss how they will carry out the evaluation phase of their plan of action based on their community assessment, nursing diagnoses, and goals set.

ACTIVITIES TO PROMOTE CRITICAL THINKING IN THE CLASSROOM

1. Using the first activity described in the textbook, take the students through a hypothetical situation using the seven steps suggested. You might try it with two very different populations (well and ill, old and young) to compare and contrast how differently the steps are conducted.

2. Select one well-functioning community program that is familiar to all students and discuss what makes it effective. What is the degree of citizen participation, leadership, and control? How does citizen involvement affect the functioning of the program? Would more citizen involvement improve the program? If so, what needs to occur to make this happen?

3. Suggest that the students participate in this activity during the term, and near the end of the term have them share the articles they found. Have each student describe the program and community health nursing involvement highlighted in their articles. Could such a program benefit the community in which the students have their clinical laboratory experience? If so, share the articles with nursing leaders in those agencies.

■ Evaluation Strategies

MULTIPLE-CHOICE QUESTIONS

1. The five major components of the nursing process are assessment, diagnosis, planning, implementation, and evaluation. The success of this process depends on a sixth component, which is:

   Client interaction
   Interaction is a necessary component of the nursing process in order for it to be effective. It is the relationship between the nurse and client that enhances reciprocal influence and exchange.

   Promoting self-care
   This is ideal but not always possible or practical with all clients.

   Data collection
   This is part of the assessment phase of the nursing process.

   Ourcome appraisal
   This is another term for evaluation—the final phase of the nursing process.

2. Community health nurses do not limit their focus to illness or health problems. They consider the client as a(n):

   Total entity
   Community health nurses look for evidence of all kinds of needs that relate to or influence a client's levels of wellness. Needs cover the whole span of the health–illness continuum and the total person, family, group, aggregate, population, or community—the total entity.

   Aggregate
   Not all clients are in the category of groups, aggregates, or populations. A client can be an individual or a family.

   Agent
   When using the epidemiological triad (Chapter 14), there are three components—host, agent, and environment. A client would be considered the host. An agent is a factor that causes or contributes to a health problem or condition.

   Community
   Not all clients are communities. They may be individuals or families.

3. Needs must be translated into which of the following to give direction and meaning to the nursing care plan or plan of action in the community?

   Goals
   The desired outcomes are described as goals and are the measurable terms into which the needs of cients must be translated in order to give direction to the nursing care plan or plan of action.

   Activities
   Activities are the steps taken to meet the objectives that flow from the goals and are the operationalization steps of the objectives.

   Outcomes
   Outcomes are the end product of the implemented plan. What is observed as an outcome is matched with stated goals. If the outcome is congruent with the goal, then the goal has been met.

   Diagnoses
   Diagnoses are used to establish needs, which guide the nurse to the planning phase.

4. When writing objectives to accomplish goals, it is most helpful if each objective:

   States a single idea and describes a specific behavior
   It is difficult to measure the objective if more than one idea and behavior are included in each.

   Is comprehensive and inclusive of desired outcomes
   Ideally, an objective states a single idea and describes one specific behavior. It would be difficult to measure the objective if more than one idea and behavior are included.

   Focuses on a nursing need
   Objectives should be client-focused needs and not nurse-focused needs.

   Is kept broad and general so it can meet the challenges of unpredictable changes
   Objectives need to be clear and specific. If circumstances change, objectives can be rewritten to accommodate the new circumstances.

5. Evaluation is an important phase of the nursing process. Its purpose is to:

Measure and judge the effectiveness of goal attainment

The purpose of evaluation is to judge value in relation to a standard and set criteria that measure the effectiveness of goal attainment.

Determine the nurse's effectiveness

The purpose of evaluation is to measure and judge the effectiveness of goal attainment, not a nurse's effectiveness. However, what may be revealed is that certain approaches or activities used to achieve goal attainment need to be modified.

Eliminate unneccessary phases in the nursing process

All phases of the nursing process are necessary.

Produce additional goals, objectives, and activities to be included in the plan

This is not the purpose of evaluation but may occur as a result of evaluation.

ESSAY QUESTIONS

1. Provide students with a community health case study that involves an aggregate. Ask them to outline steps in the nursing process and identify appropriate nursing activities to promote aggregate wellness.

2. Describe how you would complete the evaluation phase of the nursing process when implementing a wellness program with an individual client and an aggregate client. Would there be a difference? Why or why not?

INDIVIDUAL OR GROUP PROJECTS

1. Assess the quality measurement and improvement system of a clinical agency with which you are familiar. Use the characteristics of a sound quality management system (page 384 in the textbook) to guide your assessment.

2. Using the same case study in essay 1, have the students identify structure-process evaluation and outcomes-evaluation strategies they will use. Discuss why each is important.

CHAPTER 20

Communities in Crisis: Disasters, Group Violence, and Terrorism

LEARNING OBJECTIVES

Upon mastery of this chapter, you should be able to:

- Describe disasters in terms of a variety of characteristics, including causation, number of casualties, scope, and intensity.

- Discuss a variety of factors contributing to a community's potential for experiencing a disaster.

- Identify the four phases of disaster management.

- Describe the role of the community health nurse in preventing, preparing for, responding to, and supporting recovery from disasters.

- Compare and contrast the most common types of group violence.

- Discuss a variety of factors contributing to a community's potential for experiencing group violence.

- Describe the role of the community health nurse in preventing and responding to group violence.

- Distinguish terrorism from other types of group violence.

- Describe the role of the community health nurse in preventing and responding to acts of terrorism.

KEY TERMS

Arson	Indirect victim
Assault and battery	Intensity
Casualty	Looting
Critical incident stress debriefing (CISD)	Lynching
	Rape
Direct victim	Refugee
Disaster	Riot
Displaced person	Scope
Gang	Terrorism
Genocide	Triage
Homicide	Violent crime

■ Teaching Strategies

CLASSROOM TEACHING STRATEGIES

1. Discuss the role that the mass media played in a national crisis and tragedy, such as the Columbine High School shootings in Littleton, Colorado; the bombing of the U.S. Navy ship *USS Cole* in Yemen; or a recent natural disaster.

2. Select a recent crisis of local, regional, national, or global proportion that all students are familiar with and discuss (a) the characteristics of the disaster (from page 392 in the textbook), (b) types of victims (from pages 392–393), (c) role of the community health nurse at the primary, secondary, and tertiary levels of prevention, and (d) how the community health nurse fits into the elements of a disaster plan (page 395).

3. Invite a representative of the local chapter of the American Red Cross to discuss their disaster response capabilities and the various roles of volunteer disaster nurses.

CLINICAL LABORATORY TEACHING STRATEGIES

1. In the community assessment that the students conduct (Chapter 18), have them try to identify a community crisis that has occurred in the past. How was the crisis managed and resolved? What were the outcomes? How might it have been managed better, using some of the crucial steps outlined in Chapter 20?

2. After completing a community assessment of the local area, have students determine what potential crisis this community may experience, such as a factory fire, flooding, or an outbreak of a communicable disease. Have the students prepare a plan to respond at each of the three levels of prevention.

3. Ask each student to develop a disaster preparedness plan with each family assigned to them in the clinical laboratory. Include such items as fire exit plans, storage of medicines, household cleaning products, poisons, emergency phone numbers, and so on.

ACTIVITIES TO PROMOTE CRITICAL THINKING IN THE CLASSROOM

1. Use the local university community as an example and ask the students to determine some of the particular host, agent, and environment factors that might increase the community's risk for having a disaster. Such factors as age of the population, stress factors, university traffic patterns, social and educational venues attracting large numbers of people—such as concerts, sporting events, and speakers—should be considered.

2. Use the case scenario given in this activity (page 405 in the textbook) and have the students verbalize the actions they would take as a class of community health nursing students.

3. Use a local high school as an example. Discuss the possible responses the school nurse might take to address the problem of gang violence at the three levels of prevention. You might ask the school nurse for the high school to speak to the class on this subject and share the actual plans. Compare her or his comments with what the students discussed before the speaker arrived.

4. Access these sites each term (keep the compiled findings from students each term) and discuss the changing statistics for natural and man-made disasters, group violence, or terrorism with the current students. How have the statistics changed? What factors have influenced the changes?

■ Evaluation Strategies

MULTIPLE-CHOICE QUESTIONS

1. A community health nurse is working with people who experienced a tornado. These people are called the:

Direct victims
Direct victims are the people who experience the event.

Indirect victims
These victims are the relatives and friends of direct victims.

Refugees
Direct victims may or may not be refugees, but all refugees are direct victims who are forced to leave their home, usually due to war, religious persecution, or political turmoil.

Displaced persons
Displaced persons are people who have to leave their homes to escape the effect of the disaster; not all direct victims are displaced persons.

2. The goal of crisis intervention is to:

Reestablish equilibrium to the lives of those involved
The stated goal of crisis intervention is to reestablish equilibrium.

Prevent the crisis altogether
This is the best approach, but some crises, such as natural disasters, cannot be prevented. They can, however, be prepared for to decrease the negative effects of the crisis as much as possible.

Involve as many people as possible in the resolution
It is important to have an adequate number of people needed to come to resolution. However, too many people involved in resolution may cause additional confusion, chaos, and unnecessary delays.

Triage clients during the recovery phase of the crisis
Triage decisions need to be made during the response phase of the disaster or crisis and not deferred until the recovery phase. Triage is an ongoing process throughout the response phase.

3. An example of a primary prevention activity for a disaster includes:

Anticipatory guidance
Anticipating how to act to save one's life in the event of a disaster is critical. Disaster drills and practicing escape plans can save lives and are part of anticipatory guidance.

Emergency assistance
This is a secondary prevention activity.

Immediate response
This is a secondary prevention activity.

Promoting community recovery
This is a tertiary prevention activity.

4. Community health nurses can intervene to prevent various types of group violence at all three levels of prevention. Examples of involvement to prevent school violence at the secondary level include:

Participating in the school's disaster response plan at the time of an episode of violence
This is an example of a secondary prevention activity.

Offering ongoing anger management and conflict resolution courses

This is an example of a primary prevention activity.

Meeting with students, faculty, and the community to support them in their grief

This is an example of a tertiary prevention activity.

Joining organizations that engage in campaigns to reduce violence

This is an example of a primary prevention activity.

5. Community health nurses can help prevent acts of group violence, such as riots and terrorism, if they:

Look and listen within their communities for antigroup sentiments and report accordingly

Community health nurses are familiar with the normal mood and sentiment in communities and are often the first professionals to recognize escalating community tension.

Act as a negotiator when groups are at odds with each other and emotions are escalating

Community health nurses should not put themselves at risk by intervening in this manner. The best action is to get help from the police and get themselves and others in the area to safety.

Investigate in depth when situations appear to be deteriorating and violence may break out

Community health nurses should not put themselves at risk by intervening in this manner. The best action is to get help from the police and get themselves and others in the area to safety.

Follow suspects of group violence, get license plate information, and report it to the police

Community health nurses should not put themselves at risk by intervening in this manner. The best action is to inform the police of any details they have without seeking out additional information and get themselves and others in the area to safety.

ESSAY QUESTIONS

1. One of your clients, the Smyth family, is planning a large family reunion to be held in a county park. Over 100 guests are anticipated, with 10 members over age 70 and 30 under the age of 20. Make several suggestions that will help your client experience this event with the least amount of stress, making it a healthy and safe event for all guests and other people enjoying the park.

2. You come upon a two-vehicle automobile crash in a rural part of your county. There are several injured people and two bystanders. Outline your actions as a community health nurse at this crisis event. Give your rationale for each action.

INDIVIDUAL OR GROUP PROJECTS

1. Using either situation given in essay question 1 or 2, have the students work in small groups and outline the community health nurse's suggestions (in essay 1) or actions (in essay 2) and rationale for each.

2. Suggest that each student survey her or his own home and develop a disaster plan. This can be discussed in class so that each student can benefit from feedback and the plan thus improved.

CHAPTER 21

The Global Community: International Health Concerns

LEARNING OBJECTIVES

Upon mastery of this chapter, you should be able to:

- Discuss the interrelationship of global health issues.
- Describe the pluralistic medical systems of the world.
- Differentiate between multilateral and bilateral agencies.
- Explain the role of non-governmental agencies.
- Describe the purpose of the World Health Organization.
- Discuss the United States Agency for International Development (USAID).
- Analyze the implications of the Health for All movement.
- Be familiar with specific global health concerns.
- Describe what is meant by the Global Burden of Disease and Disability-Adjusted Life Year.
- Differentiate between eradication, elimination, and control of communicable disease.
- Identify new and emerging diseases.
- Increase awareness of the role of the global nurse.
- Summarize global nursing opportunities.

KEY TERMS

Bilateral agencies
Chronic disease
Disability-Adjusted
 Life Year (DALY)
Eradication, elimination,
 and control of
 communicable disease
Global Burden of
 Disease (GBD)
Global nursing
Health for All
Integrated management
 of childhood illness
 (IMCI)
Multilateral agencies

New and emerging
 diseases
Non-governmental
 organizations (NGOs)
Pluralistic medical
 systems
Primary health care
Private voluntary
 organizations (PVOs)
United States Agency for
 International
 Development (USAID)
World Bank (WB)
World Health
 Organization (WHO)

■ Teaching Strategies

CLASSROOM TEACHING STRATEGIES

1. Inquire whether any students in class have personal experience with global health agencies, both governmental and non-governmental, and ask them to share their experiences. What were the services provided or activities in which they were engaged? (Some students may be from refugee or immigrant families, and some U.S.-born students may have heard of CARE packages or collected change for UNICEF at Halloween.)

2. Discuss three governmental global health agencies (World Health Organization, World Bank, and the United States Agency for International Development) and compare their roles with various non-governmental orgainzations.

3. Discuss the 30 leading causes of death worldwide in 1990 (Display 21-7, page 415 in the textbook). Did the students think that HIV would be last on the list? Did they think measles would be on the list? Did they think drowning was in the top 20 causes of death? As another activity, prior to assigning this chapter, suggest that the students list what they believe are the top 30 causes of death in the world. Begin your discussion from their list.

4. Invite a community health nurse who has served in the Peace Corp or as a missionary to speak to the class regarding her or his observations and experiences while involved in global health improvement.

CLINICAL LABORATORY TEACHING STRATEGIES

1. If the community health nursing students are providing care to immigrant or refugee families as a part of their clinical laboratory experience, have them include the type of health care the family

received in their native country in the family assessments. Discuss the quality and quantity of the services available to these families prior to arriving in the U.S. How much do you feel the services relate to the health of the family members today? Perhaps some of the nursing students are from immigrant or refugee families or are international students. Ask them to share their own family's experiences with their native country's health care system.

2. Have the community health nursing students explore the laboratory services of the health department serving the local community. Ask the department head to discuss the types of diseases they see and how the diseases have changed in the last 10 years. What has contributed to the changes? How much of the change can be attributed to immigration and/or an increase in international travel?

ACTIVITIES TO PROMOTE CRITICAL THINKING IN THE CLASSROOM

1. Have the students bring these data to class and facilitate a discussion on the differences discovered and identified contributing factors.

2. Using the morbidity statistics for the same countries, discuss the diferences among the countries and possible contributing factors.

3. Discuss the health care system in each of the countries in activity 1 and 2. How do the systems, their funding, organization, and size contribute to the mortality and morbidity statistics for the different countries?

4. Discuss measles as a leading cause of death in the world. Suggest that the class work in three or four groups and devise a plan for eradication. Allow about 20 minutes for this activity, then have the students compare the plans and decide on one "best" plan. Do the countries with the highest rate of measles have the resources (professional and para-professional personnel and money) needed to implement such a plan? If not, how will the group proceed?

5. Have the students search the Internet and find current information about the "Health for All" movement. How is it progressing? What are some of the major barriers if it is not progressing? Is there anything the U.S. can do to improve the progress?

6. Discuss the newspaper articles collected throughout the term by the community health nursing students. What role is politics playing in the health issues addressed in the articles?

■ Evaluation Strategies

MULTIPLE-CHOICE QUESTIONS

1. As a community health nurse, it is important for you to know the World Health Organization's (WHO) mission. It is in existence to:

Promote health on a global basis by directing and coordinating international health work
This describes the mission of the WHO.

Collaborate in health development and make the world "free from poverty"
This describes the mission of the World Bank.

Serve as an independent agency providing economic and humanitarian assistance overseas
This describes the United States Agency for International Development (USAID). WHO serves all member countries worldwide, not just overseas.

Represent the global interests and concerns of the nursing profession
This describes the role of the International Council of Nurses (ICN).

2. The Declaration of Alma-Ata is important to global public health because it represents:

A formal document written by 134 nations in 1978 to achieve "health for all"
This declaration represents the work of these countries during a WHO/UNICEF conference in 1978 to achieve primary health care for all.

The beginning of the Carter Center's work in disease prevention and agriculture
The Carter Center was founded in 1986 and is not related to the work at Alma-Ata.

Participatory development activities, working in partnership with voluntary organizations
This describes the work of the United States Agency for International Development (USAID).

Alliance building and communicating best practices for global health development
This describes the Global Health Council, which is a leading private, voluntary, American non-governmental organization.

3. Communicable disease is a global health concern; therefore, there is a primary goal to eradicate communicable diseases worldwide. This would include:

The interruption of transmission and reservoir of infection so that no further cases occur anywhere

Eradication is an ambitious and expensive goal and has occurred with smallpox in 1977 and is under way with other diseases such as poliomyelitis, guinea worm, leprosy, and measles so that we may see many diseases eradicated early in the 21st century.

The interruption of a disease in a limited, defined geographic area

This describes elimination and is not as ambitious an achievement as eradication.

Reducing the incidence and/or prevalence of communicable diseases

This describes control and is not as broad an achievement as elimination or eradication.

The establishment of primary health care services for all people on the globe

This represents the goal of Alma-Ata as first defined in 1978—"health for all."

4. There is currently a worldwide tuberculosis epidemic. The statistics are grim, and the picture of the disease looks like this:

TB kills 2 to 3 million people each year.

This is the number of global deaths from TB each year.

Someone in the world is newly infected with TB every hour.

If this were true, TB would be under control. Someone is newly infected every second.

Nearly 10% of the world's population is infected with TB each year.

Nearly 1% is infected each year; if it were 10%, in 10 years everyone would be infected.

Half of the TB cases per year occur in Eastern Europe.

250,000 cases of TB occur each year in Eastern Europe, and there are 7 to 8 million new cases worldwide each year.

5. Community health nurses are important in the global health arena because:

There are more community health nurses than any other professional group providing health services to people everywhere.

This is true; they are involved with and provide a wider range of services in multiple settings than any other health care professional.

It is through community health nurses that the larger number of physicians do their work.

Community health nurses are in greater numbers on a global scale than any other professional group, including physicians.

They work for lower wages than other professional groups.

Many community health nurses work voluntarily, as do other professional groups serving the global community. Pay scales are not a major issue in global health; most participate for the experience and the humanitarian good will.

They are the only group that people in other countries trust and allow to help.

This is not true. Volunteer health care professionals from many other countries work around the world in global health care. All are accepted by the people they serve on the basis of their commitment to social action programs and acceptance of cross-cultural opportunities.

ESSAY QUESTIONS

1. You are the only professional health care provider working with the native population of a small island in the Pacific. There is an outbreak of a diarrheal disease on the far side of the island, 6 miles away, where 1000 inhabitants live (one third of the island's population). You are located on the other side of the island where the remaining inhabitants live. How would you handle this crisis until additional help arrives in 2 days?

2. Select one of the 30 leading causes of death worldwide and suggest strategies that could be used to eradicate, eliminate, and control the selected cause of death.

INDIVIDUAL OR GROUP PROJECTS

1. Using Display 21-7 (page 415) with the 30 leading causes of death worldwide in 1990 as a starting point, explore the ordering of the top 30 causes 10 or more years later, in the year 2000, 2001, 2002, etc. Which diseases or conditions are no longer on the list? Which have moved up? What has contributed to the change and the ranking for the year you researched? Are there new causes on the list?

2. Currently, tuberculosis is a worldwide epidemic killing 2 to 3 million people a year. It also is a problem in your local community. Explore the current efforts in your community to eradicate, eliminate, and/or control TB. What do you think needs to be done to improve your community's efforts?

UNIT V

The Family as Client

CHAPTER 22

Theoretical Bases for Promoting Family Health

LEARNING OBJECTIVES

Upon mastery of this chapter, you should be able to:

- Analyze changing definitions of family.

- Discuss characteristics all families have in common.

- Identify five attributes that help explain how families function as social systems.

- Discuss how a family's culture influences its values, behaviors, prescribed roles, and distributions of power.

- Compare and contrast the variety of structures that make up families.

- Describe the functions of a family.

- Identify the stages of the family life cycle and the developmental tasks of a family as it grows.

- Analyze the role of the community health nurse in promoting the health of the family unit.

KEY TERMS

Adoptive family	Group-network family
Blended family	Homeless family
Cohabitating couples	Intrarole functioning
Commune family	Kin-network
Commuter family	Multigenerational family
Contemporary family	Nontraditional family
Energy exchange	Nuclear-dyad family
Family	Nuclear family
Family culture	Primary relationship
Family functioning	Roles
Family map	Single-adult family
Family structure	Single-parent family
Family system boundary	Stepfamily
Foster families	Traditional family
Gangs	Wider family
Group-marriage family	

■ Teaching Strategies

CLASSROOM TEACHING STRATEGIES

1. Discuss several popular television situation comedies or dramas. Ask students to identify the family structures depicted in these shows. Which are traditional and which are nontraditional (use Table 22-1. Page 434)? How well do these TV families fulfill the functions and tasks as depicted in Table 22-2, page 440?

2. Suggest that students volunteer to describe their own family structure using the appropriate tables from Chapter 22. Discuss the differences shared.

3. Throughout the course, have students collect impressions of traditional and nontraditional family functioning from community health nurses practicing in a variety of settings. Compare and contrast the various nurses' views.

CLINICAL LABORATORY TEACHING STRATEGIES

1. Have each student assess assigned families in relation to being a traditional or nontraditional family. Share this information among peers. What percent are traditional American families? What percent are nontraditional American families? Were any of the families new to the American culture? If so, how did their family structure compare? How many are nuclear families? Did any of the percentages surprise the students? Which percentages and why?

2. Have the students repeat the above activity with their clients over the age of 65. Ask the older adults about the family structure they grew up in. Have the percentages or types of family structures changed using an older population? If so, what might be the reasons?

ACTIVITIES TO PROMOTE CRITICAL THINKING IN THE CLASSROOM

1. Use this activity in the classroom by dividing the class into small groups and follow through with the various questions.

2. Select two families that are familiar to the class (families from the clinical laboratory, a TV family, such as "Everybody Loves Raymond," "Malcomb in the Middle," or "The Simpsons", or two of the student's own families) and answer questions a through e. This can be a fun activity especially if a TV family is chosen.

3. Again, draw on the students' experiences to select blended families to discuss. The family can come from the clinical laboratory or be volunteered from among the students' own families. Discuss the three questions in this activity.

4. Gay and lesbian couples often seek parenting opportunities. Use the questions in this activity and facilitate a general discussion on this topic. The discussion would be more lively if the class is divided on the issue. If they aren't, you can play "devil's advocate" and take the opposite stance for sake of discussion.

5. Suggest that the students engage in this activity at the beginning of the term. Near the middle of the term discuss the students' findings and focus the discussion on the two questions in this activity.

■ Evaluation Strategies

MULTIPLE-CHOICE QUESTIONS

1. Which of the following best describes the most current definition of family?

The family is who the client says it is
Family structure is unique, and currently whoever makes up a family in any particular household is considered by them a family. This is regardless of bloodlines or legal arrangements.

Only persons who are related by a common bloodline
This is no longer a popular definition of family. It was popular in years past.

Persons who are involved in the same social groups in a community
This does not define family. It better describes groups of common interest.

Persons who live in close proximity to one another
This may or may not define family. Many people live close together due to the architectural configuration of housing, but the people involved do not consider themselves a family.

2. There are universal characteristics of families that include:

Cultural values and rules
These two characteristics are shared by all families and are unique within each family.

System boundaries that are closed
Family boundaries are semipermeable, providing protection and preservation of family unity and autonomy while also allowing selective linkage with external associations.

Remaining in one stage of their life cycle
All families moves through stages in their life cycle. They are not static—they are dynamic.

No particular structure, as families are dynamic
All families have structure, albeit different from other families, but a defined structure.

3. Families demonstrate attributes as social systems. The following attributes help to explain how families function:

Families exchange energy with their environment.
Family boundaries are semipermeable, and as open systems they exchange materials or information with their environment.

Family members are independent.
All the members of a family are interdependent, not independent. Each member's actions affect the other members.

Families remain the same and generally do not adapt.
Families are adaptive, equilibrium-seeking systems and never stay the same.

Family structures are not goal directed.
As social systems they are goal directed. They exist for a purpose, and in order to fulfill this purpose they must work toward goals.

4. A family's culture influences its own unique values. An example of explicitly stated values is the following:

"Family problems stay within the family."
This describes a family's values and leads to a rule for operation. Such a value may be operationalized with "Don't tell anyone about our problems."

"Bring me the milk since you are near the refrigerator."
This statement does not depict an explicitly stated value, it is simply a request.

"Dinner is ready and is on the stove."
This statement does not depict an explicitly stated value, it is simply an announcement.

"Report cards come out on Friday."
This statement does not depict an explicitly stated value, it is simply an announcement.

5. In what way does a nuclear dyad differ from a nuclear family?

The nuclear dyad family is childless or the children are launched.
A nuclear dyad consists of two people—male and female—living as a couple who either have no children or whose children are launched.

The children in a nuclear dyad family are infants and not walking yet.
A nuclear family is made up of two people—male and female—and their children living together. There are no children living at home in a nuclear dyad family.

The children in a nuclear dyad family are of school age.
A nuclear family is made up of two people—male and female—and their children living together. There are no children living at home in a nuclear dyad family.

A nuclear dyad family is multigenerational.
A nuclear dyad family is made up of two people— male and female—and is not multigenerational.

6. Which of the following is an example of a nontraditonal family?

A homeless family
This family remains nontraditional; however, there are more and more families who are homeless. Drugs, alcohol, increased cost of living and housing, and divorce all contribute to this new nontraditional family.

A nuclear dyad
This is a traditional family—a male and female living as a couple.

A divorced family
Over 50% of all marriages end in divorce today, and it has been a part of society for years. Because it has been so common for so many years, it has become a traditional form of family.

A nuclear family
This is a traditional family—a male and female living together with their children.

ESSAY QUESTIONS

1. The Jones' have been married for six years. They have 4 children. Two (aged 16 and 13) are from Mrs. Jones' first marriage. One (Age 9) is from Mr. Jones' first marriage. Their 3 year old is from their union. Using the family characteristics outlined in this chapter, describe the type of family and the appropriate stage-critical family developental tasks you as a student community health nurse would include in a family assessment or in providing anticipatory guidance to this family.

2. "Gangs" are considered a nontraditional family. Identify how a community health nurse could work effectively with youth at risk for gang involvement at the primary, secondary or teriary level of prevention to promote an individual member's health.

INDIVIDUAL OR GROUP PROJECTS

1. Have each student keep a journal of their own family interactions during the duration of the course and note areas that could be worked on to have a healthier family life.

2. Have the students select a family they are familiar with and describe how they meet the six family functions described in Chapter 22 on pages 436–438.

CHAPTER 23

Assessment of Families

LEARNING OBJECTIVES

Upon mastery of this chapter, you should be able to:

- Describe the effect of family health on individual health and community health.

- Describe individual and group characteristics of a healthy family.

- Identify five family health practice guidelines.

- Describe three conceptual frameworks that can be used to assess a family.

- Describe the 12 major assessment categories for families.

- List the five basic principles the community health nurse should follow when assessing family health.

KEY TERMS

Conceptual framework	Genogram
Developmental framework	Interactional framework
Eco-map	Social network support map
Family health	Strengthening
Family nursing	Structural-functional framework

■Teaching Strategies

CLASSROOM TEACHING STRATEGIES

1. Provide the students with the five case studies in this chapter (Displays 23-1 to 23-5 on pages 450–453), or other case studies you might choose, and have the students identify some healthy characteristics and unhealthy characteristics of these families. Describe how the health or illness of the families could influence the health of their communities.

2. Have a school nurse or another community health nurse discuss with the class how family relationships and family health practices influence a child's ability to perform academically and to interact effectively with peers.

CLINICAL LABORATORY TEACHING STRATEGIES

1. Ask students to use the family assessment tools in the text to study a family or families as part of their clinical laboratory experience. Have the students share their assessments with the class or place them in a journal for the faculty member to review.

2. Ask students to complete an ecomap and/or genogram of one of the families they visit in their clinical laboratory experience. Have the students share their ecomap or genogram with the class or place them in a journal for the faculty member to review.

ACTIVITIES TO PROMOTE CRITICAL THINKING IN THE CLASSROOM

1. Suggest that this activity be conducted in class between pairs of students. After they complete the questions in this activity, ask them to share some of their findings with the whole class. Did the students find more similarities or more differences?

2. Ask for a student volunteer to share her or his genogram and allow the class to look for family trends or traits. Ask the student whether she or he has any new insights about the family? If time permits, do this activity with more students and compare famiy findings.

3. Ask for a student volunteer to share her or his social support network map or grid with the class. Ask for feedback from the class and listen to the student's plan to enhance her or his network based on her or his own observations or class feedback. Perhaps review several other neworks to see the variety among the students. If there is a lot of variety among the students, how might the networks of clients in the community vary?

4. Ask a student to bring a completed family assessment form to class. Place it on a transparency with identifying data removed for confidentiality. As a class, work on determining as many nursing interventions as possible that could be used to promote this family's health.

■ Evaluation Strategies

MULTIPLE-CHOICE QUESTIONS

1. An ecomap is a useful tool for community health nurses because it:

   Diagrams the connections between the family and other systems
   An ecomap diagrams a family's relatonships to its external environment. Lines are drawn to indicate connections to other systems, arrows signify the direction of energy or flow of resources, and absence of lines indicates a lack of connections.

   Diagrams family relationships over three or more generations
   This defines a genogram, which is useful to show family patterns and traits to the nurse and provides insight into the larger family to the current family members.

   Charts the ecological system of a family's neighborhood
   This is not the purpose of an ecomap.

   Provides directions for gathering data about neighborhoods
   This is not the purpose of an ecomap.

2. In the Levels of Family Functioning Model by Tapia, the family in childhood (Level II) is:

   Slightly above survival level with limited ability to trust
   The Level II family is at a higher level of functioning than the chaotic Level I family. They remain disorganized and have limited ability to trust. However, the family functions lower than the Level III family (a fairly normal family with more than its share of problems).

   An average family with more than its share of problems
   This describes the Level III family.

   A well family functioning independently
   This describes the Level IV family.

   Very chaotic and barely surviving
   This describes the Level I family.

3. The nurse working with the Beck family (depicted in Display 23-1 on page 450) is an example of how the nurse:

   Works with the family as a collective whole
   In the example cited, the nurse works with the family as a whole, not with individuals, to change behaviors. The family participates in the activities to achieve family goals.

   Starts where the family is
   This is inherent in the nurse's work with all families. It is depicted in Display 23-2 on page 451 with the Kegler family.

   Adapts intervention according to family stage of development
   This is inherent in the nurse's work with all families. It is depicted in Display 23-3 on page 451 with the Roberts family.

   Recognizes the validity of family structure variations
   This is inherent in the nurse's work with all families. It is depicted in Display 23-4 on page 452 with the James Cutler and Brian Hoag family.

4. How does an interactional framework describe the family?

   By looking at the interacting personalities between family members
   The interactional framework portrays the family unit as a union of interacting personalities. It describes the family in terms of its internal relationships, emphasizing communications, roles, conflict, coping patterns, and decision-making processes.

   From a life-cycle perspective
   An interactional framework does not consider the life-cycle perspective of individuals or families.

   In terms of the characteristics of a healthy family
   The characteristics of a healthy family are broader and refer to individual development and linking with the broader community, which the interactional framework does not address.

   As a social system relating to other social systems
   An interactional framework does not consider the family's interaction with its external environment.

5. When a community health nurse is planning to conduct an accurate family assessment on an assigned family, it is best to:

   Make several visits and accumulate data from all family members
   Making an accurate family assessment takes time. It is better to keep notes from several visits with the family and observe the family as a group during some family activity.

   Use quantitative data only to maintain and preserve objectivity
   The nurse should collect both qualtitative and qualitative data, which will provide a rich family assessment.

Interview one family member to avoid confusion and repeated information

This will give a one-sided view of family data. It is best to interview all family members over time.

Use a checklist format and complete the tool in the family's presence

The nurse should not use obtrusive questionnaire techniques or take notes in the family's presence.

ESSAY QUESTIONS

1. Using the data collection method in Table 23-1 on page 455, assess your own family, including the twelve assessment categories.

2. Using two of the five case studies in this chapter, assess them for their level of health using the six characteristics for a healthy family found on pages 447 to 448.

INDIVIDUAL OR GROUP PROJECTS

1. Ask the students to assess their own families through the use of a genogram and share them verbally with the class. Each student should bring samples of family photos and identify ages and causes of death aong deceased family members. Do any specific patterns emerge? Discuss observations. This activity takes time and is best conducted in clinical laboratory groups of 8 to 12. It is also a useful tool for students to get to know one another even after being in classes together for years.

2. Among a specified number of students or in one clinical laboratory group, assess each assigned client family according to the Tapia Model presented in this chapter on pages 456 and 459. In what levels do most families function? What does this mean for the role of the nurse and types of services provided?

CHAPTER 24

Planning, Intervening, and Evaluating Health Care to Families

LEARNING OBJECTIVES

Upon mastery of this chapter, you should be able to:

- Describe the components of the nursing process as applied to enhancing family health.

- Identify the steps in a successful family health intervention.

- Discuss the two foci of family health visits: education and health promotion.

- List at least six specific safety measures the community health nurse should take when traveling to and/or making a home visit.

- Describe useful activities and actions when intervening on family health visits.

- Describe three types of evaluations that are necessary following family health intervention.

KEY TERMS

Home visit	Outcome evaluation
Mutual goals	Referral
Nursing bag	Resource directory

■ Teaching Strategies

CLASSROOM TEACHING STRATEGIES

1. Role play making a home visit with students taking the roles of community health nurse and various family members. Use the Guidelines for Making Home Visits in Display 24-2 on page 474 as a guide. Use the five family scenarios in Chapter 23 as the families visited.

2. Discuss safety precautions you would recommend for students when traveling in the community during their clinical laboratory experiences. Are there differences in preparing to travel in rural versus urban neighborhoods? Include additional recommendations based on your knowledge of the community.

CLINICAL LABORATORY TEACHING STRATEGIES

1. After the clinical laboratory assignments have been made, suggest that the students review the client family charts or referrals and then go around the student group and role play setting up the first family health visit and entering the home based on family information in the chart or referral. Having the students practice using the telephone to introduce themselves, stating the agency name, sounding assertive yet friendly, and repeating the same to get into the home helps to give them the support they may need for this "nursing without walls" experience.

2. Have each student write up at least one family contract to use with an assigned family (see sample on page 481). Share them during a clinical conference to give the group ideas for additional family contracts.

ACTIVITIES TO PROMOTE CRITICAL THINKING IN THE CLASSROOM

1. Discuss the students' observations of one another on family health visits in the home. To move the discussion quickly, ask for positive things the observer saw the peer do. Ask the observers what they saw that the student conducting the visit missed.

2. Ask the students to share what they observed when they went on family health visits with staff nurses from the clinical laboratory agency or from another agency with community health nurses in the community. Ask how the students will incorporate some of the practices into their own home visits.

3. Continue the discussion on safety in the community by including campus safety, safety practices at home or in a dormitory, out shopping, or traveling to clinical laboratory sites for other nursing courses. Are safety practices different depending on the setting? Should they be?

4. Have the students go to the Internet and look for current nursing articles based on using the Olds Model—intensive home visits to high-risk families—and bring them to class for discussion. Do any agencies in the community use this model in their practice? If so, explore their program and share it with the class. Suggest that a staff member from an agency using the Olds Model present their program to the class.

▪ Evaluation Strategies

MULTIPLE-CHOICE QUESTIONS

USE THE FOLLOWING SCENARIO FOR QUESTIONS 1 to 3.

You are a student community health nurse and are about to make your first home visit to a family based on a referral from the hospital where the high-risk infant you are about to visit was born 6 days ago. The mother, Jonquil, is 17 years old, and the newborn, Herbie, weighed 5 pounds, 11 ounces at birth. Your plans are to assess the family and home environment and provide anticipatory guidance.

1. Jonquil sleepily answers the door after you ring the bell and knock several times. She is not happy to see you but lets you in. She tells you to sit down; she gets Herbie and places him in your arms, then sits across the room and turns on the TV. You are surprised by her actions, but the first thing you say to her is:

"You must be very tired caring for a newborn baby."
It is always best to acknowledge a client's feelings, and from your observations and referral information, being fatigued 6 days after having a baby is very possible.

"I wasn't planning to hold the baby. You should hold him, you are the mother."
This is not the best way to respond to the mother or the first comment, but holding the baby gives you an opportunity to role model infant interaction and caring and assess his cleanliness and clothing appropriateness. However, you may want to say that you would like to wash your hands before holding Herbie. This gives you an additional opportunity to teach and assess another room when you wash your hands.

"I would like to talk to you, and I would like to have the TV turned off."
This might be something you would say after a few moments of introductory conversation. It would be best to ask Jonquil to turn the TV down as

you are having trouble hearing her rather than turning it off—it might be her favorite program that she missed by oversleeping. You will win her favor with this approach better than by asking her to turn off the TV.

"How do you feel being a mother at 17?"
This might be information you want to gather, but asking it directly sounds like a put-down. There are better ways to obtain this information.

2. You chat with Jonquil and ask her if you can do a newborn assessment on Herbie. She has reservations about this, but you explain that doing this gives you an opportunity to:

Show her interesting things about her baby's development at 1 week of age.
This approach is more positive and educational than one that depicts the nurse as an inspector looking for something Jonquil did wrong.

Check how well she has been caring for the baby.
No one wants to hear this, especially a 17-year-old new mother.

See if Herbie looks like other newborn babies.
This is not something you would say, but as you assess the baby you are looking for normal parameters.

Assure the hospital that she is a good mother.
You will report back to the hospital on the referral to complete the referral cycle, but this is not the purpose of the visit, and you may have negative information to report to the hospital.

3. During the assessment you find that Herbie looks healthy, and Jonquil seems very interested with several questions. One question she asks is whether you are going to see her again. Your best response is:

"I can come as often as you like—it depends on what we want to accomplish together."
This represents a mutual approach, giving power to the client and hints at accomplishing things together on subsequent visits.

"Herbie looks good, and one or two visits more are all that is needed."
This might be all the visits you actually make, but to say it like this is closed-ended and nurse focused and does not promote open communication between the client and the nurse.

"The agency limits the number of visits I can make; I will let you know."
The nurse has more control over the number of visits than this response implies, unless the visit is part of a special and very limited program. Even then it would not be phrased this way.

"I can come weekly for the next 16 weeks, and then a staff nurse will visit."

This answer reflects the student semester (9 weeks if on a quarter system) and may be the way clients are handled in the clinical laboratory agency, where staff nurses continue with some clients after students leave. However, this is not how it should be presented to the client. "Sixteen visits and then a new nurse will continue" sounds overwhelming. Very few clients receive this much service from public health agencies.

4. You are making a family health visit, and an older relative who is visiting has been drinking and becomes verbally abusive and increasingly loud. As the nurse it is best to:

Terminate the visit and make plans for another visit.

This is the best choice. It appears the problem is escalating, and your safety should always come first.

Continue the visit with caution.

It appears the problem is escalating, and your safety should always come first. Continuing puts you and possibly the other family members at risk.

Suggest the relative go in another room and take a nap.

It appears the problem is escalating, and your safety should always come first. Making such a suggestion may agitate the relative and make a deteriorating situation worse.

Ask the sober family members to take the visitor home.

It appears the problem is escalating, and your safety should always come first. Making such a suggestion may agitate the relative and make a deteriorating situation worse.

5. A client you are visiting asks you to take her shopping to purchase some of the food items she needs for her diet. You respond by saying:

You are unable to do this but will help her find a way to get to the store.

This is the best choice as it clarifies what you can and cannot do as a nurse, and one of the things you can do is help her find transportation. You will not always be there to assist her. If you drove the client to the store, you would not be empowering her and you would be setting a precedent you will not be able to maintain with other families in the future.

You are too busy and are going in a different direction from the store.

Part of this is true, and part is probably a fabrication. It is best to be honest and help the client find transportation she can rely on when she needs it.

This is not the role of a nurse and she will have to find other transportation.

This is not a very warm, friendly, or helpful response. A community health nurse should be able to be more helpful.

She can start her diet with the foods she has in the house and shop next week.

This is not a very helpful response. A community health nurse should be able to be more helpful and meet the client's needs and not make judgments or decisions for the client.

ESSAY QUESTIONS

1. Mrs. Roselle is a 79-year-old widow who lives alone in a small home on the outskirts of town. She needs assistance to remember to take her five medications for hypertension and congestive heart failure. Develop a family contract that addressess this issue.

2. Express your feelings as you enter community health nursing. Share your concerns, doubts, and fears. Develop a plan to overcome apprehensions.

INDIVIDUAL OR GROUP PROJECTS

1. Using the flow sheet for a high-risk infant on pages 479 to 480 as a model, have small groups of students develop flow sheets for high-risk prenatal and postpartum clients, well infants and children, healthy older adults, and individuals with specific chronic diseases. Use these tools for student charting if the agency does expect the students to chart home visits, or with agencies that do not have a charting system in place, such as neighborhood centers, senior centers, or senior housing developments.

2. Review some of the family charts in the clinical laboratory agency for the evaluation component. Is it there? Is it well developed? Does it provide useful information for the next nurse? Does it flow from the interventions and guide the nurse to new planning? What should be done differently to make the evaluation component stronger and more useful? Do this as a clinical group or individually to improve your own caregiving and charting.

CHAPTER 25

Families in Crisis: Domestic Violence and Abuse

LEARNING OBJECTIVES

Upon mastery of this chapter, you should be able to:

- Explain the difference between developmental crises and situational crises and give several examples of each within families.

- Discuss strategies to prevent the impact of a situational crisis and a developmental crisis at each level of prevention.

- Discuss the global incidence and prevalence of family violence.

- Describe how the U.S. has historically responded to family violence.

- Describe three main categories of family violence.

- Identify characteristics of five forms of abuse against infants, children, and adolescents.

- Describe the "cycle of violence" seen in partner/spousal abuse.

- Explain the types of mistreatment common to the elderly.

- Describe the role of a community health nurse with families in crisis at each level of prevention.

- Use the steps of the nursing process to outline nursing actions in developmental and situational crises.

KEY TERMS

Battered child syndrome	Incest
Child abuse	Intrafamilial sexual abuse
Coping	Mandated reporters
Corporal punishment	Munchausen syndrome by proxy
Crisis theory	Neglect
Cycle of violence	Pedophile
Dating violence	Physical abuse
Developmental crisis	Rape
Domestic violence	Sexual abuse
Elder abuse	Sexual exploitation
Emotional abuse	Shaken baby syndrome
Family crisis	Situational crisis
Family violence	Spousal abuse
Homicide	Suicide

■ Teaching Strategies

CLASSROOM TEACHING STRATEGIES

1. Discuss the incidence and prevalence of family violence in your university community. Suggest that a counselor from student health services talk to the students and give a broad picture of family violence on campus and how to recognize potentially abusive situations when dating. Suggest that the counselor review the health services on campus for student use and student referrals.

2. Discuss family violence and cultural differences. If some students are first-generation Americans or from families with strong ties to another culture, ask them to share child-rearing practices, the view of women, and the view of the aged in their culture. How have these practices changed over the years and after experiencing American culture?

CLINICAL LABORATORY TEACHING STRATEGIES

1. Review the forms used by various community agencies to document physical and sexual abuse when a person is seen in the emergency department. Review them for several reasons: to educate the students on what to look for in a potentially abused client, so they will know how thorough the examination is and can share this with clients, and to critique the data that are gathered on the forms for completeness.

2. During a clinical conference, discuss the various types of abuse and neglect observed among assigned clients visited and cared for during the term. What are some of the problems the clients have in common? What contributes to these situations? How can the community health nurse prevent them at the primary level of prevention?

ACTIVITIES TO PROMOTE CRITICAL THINKING IN THE CLASSROOM

1. Ask the students to share some of the major events in their lives, such as an illness, injury, marriage, birth of children, and so on. Ask them whether the event was a situational crisis or a developmental crisis. Have them give rationale for each type of crisis. Suggest the students identify the primary, secondary, and tertiary levels of prevention to prevent the impact of their situational and developmental crises.

2. Use an example of a developmental crisis from the clinical laboratory experience. How might the community health nurse have improved the outcome if involved with this family at the primary level of prevention?

3. Discuss school violence using some well-known cases, such as Columbine High School in Littleton, Colorado, or local episodes of childhood violence that have occurred more recently. What is the nurse's role on an interprofessional team to prevent such occurrences at the primary level of prevention? What is the nurse's role at the secondary and tertiary levels of prevention? Invite a school nurse to be a speaker in class and describe her or his role during an act of childhood violence in a school she or he serves.

4. Select some situational crises that have been brought to the public's attention from around the world through the media. Discuss them in class. How could a community health nurse have intervened successfully at all levels of prevention in the crises?

5. Use examples of women and children from the clinical laboratory experience who have suffered from family violence and describe how the community health nurse can provide assistance at all levels of prevention. Invite a speaker to class from children's services, a foster parent, or a police officer to discuss her or his role in family violence.

6. During the term, have the students share the latest information regarding family violence that they have uncovered while using the Internet. Tie their findings into the topic you are currently discussing. For example, whether you are teaching epidemiology, the legislative process, or roles of the community health nurse, current information on family violence can be woven into the content.

■ Evaluation Strategies

MULTIPLE-CHOICE QUESTIONS

1. A developmental crisis is:

   Precipitated by a life transition
   A developmental crisis is defined as a transitional event in a person's normal growth and development that is disruptive and stressful.

   Sudden in onset and unexpected
   Developmental crises, as a rule, do not occur suddenly; they are slow transitions into new stages that lead to new events. Even the aging, illness, or death of a grandparent or parent is a developmental expectation. However, the actual event may occur suddenly.

   Precipitated by a hazardous event
   This describes how a situational crisis may occur.

   An externally imposed accident
   This describes one way a situational crisis may occur.

2. Primary situational crisis prevention involves:

   Meeting basic needs through anticipatory guidance and education
   This describes primary situational crisis prevention. The goal is to prevent the incident from occurring by improving the environment where situational crises may occur, such as in dysfunctional families or unsafe physical environments.

   Early detection and response when a situational crisis occurs
   This describes secondary situational crisis prevention.

   Rehabilitation and restoration of a victim's life
   This describes tertiary situational crisis prevention.

   The work of professionals during the situational crisis
   This describes tertiary situational crisis prevention.

3. The history of family or domestic violence:

   Is not new—it has occurred in most countries for centuries
   The history of family and domestic violence is long. It is only fairly recently in history (1900) that groups have become concerned and begun to do something about family violence.

   Is new as a result of our fast-paced technological society
   The history of family and domestic violence is long. It is brought to attention in urban areas where

*people live more closely, but occurs in all
segments of society—rural and urban.*

Occurs mostly in the urbanized areas of the United
States

*It is brought to the attention of officials more
frequently today than in yesteryear, especially in
urban areas where more people live, but it occurs
throughout the world—in urban, rural, and
remote areas.*

Is decreasing in industrialized countries in the world

*It is brought to attention in urban areas where
people live more closely, but has been occurring
in all segments of society in all countries with no
signs of decreasing; in fact, it is increasing.*

4. Child neglect is a common form of child abuse.
Which of the following situation constitutes a form
of child neglect?

Fifteen-year-old Lucy misses school once a week to
watch her 1-year-old sister while her mother
works.

*This is a form of educational neglect for Lucy. The
mother should make other arrangements for the
1-year-old.*

Six-year-old Sam plays in the yard with just a
sweater on when it is only 55 degrees outside.

*This may be appropriate based on how hard and
long he is playing—he may be comfortable.*

Nine-year-old Bobby misses school two or three
times a month due to asthma attacks.

*Although Bobby is missing a number of days of
school, he has a legitimate excuse.*

Fourteen-year-old Jennifer watches her next door
neighbor's 2-year-old every Saturday.

Fourteen is an appropriate and legal age to babysit.

5. Which of the following statements about abuse in
families is a myth?

Women who accept battering are mentally ill.

*The percentage of battered women who are
mentally ill is the same as in the general
population; however, they have low self-esteem
and a damaged spirit.*

Family violence occurs across all incomes.

*This is a true statement—no income group is
immune to family violence.*

Domestic violence has no gender or sexual
boundaries.

*This is a true statement—no gender or sexual
boundaries protect from family violence.*

Many abusers do not drink or use durgs.

*This is a true statement—drinking or using drugs
may escalate abuse, but abuse also occurs in
families who do not use drugs or drink.*

6. A community health nurse is designated as a
"mandated reporter." This means:

The nurse must report suspected abuse and neglect.

*The abuse or neglect simply needs to be suspected
in order for the nurse to report. In most states
the nurse can receive a jail sentence and a fine
for not reporting suspected abuse.*

The nurse must witness abuse and neglect before
being mandated to report.

*The abuse or neglect simply has to be suspected in
order to report. The nurse (or others) may never
witness the actual abusive event, but they can
often see the resulting damage.*

The nurse mandates that battered women report the
abuse.

*This is not the meaning of mandated reporter.
Battered women often need to be encouraged
strongly, several times, before they report abuse,
and many never do.*

An agency community health nurse is the staff
member who reports abuse to the state.

*This is not the meaning of mandated reporter. Each
nurse follows through with reporting abuse and
neglect cases she or he suspects according to the
community's laws. A social worker from
children's services follows up on the report. At
times, if the nurse knows the family, she or he
may make a shared visit with the social worker.*

7. Munchausen syndrome by proxy may be suspected
if a child:

Experiences "seizures" only when a parent is
present, not when a third party is present

*This would be a "red flag" for this syndrome if it
were occurring in a child you were caring for in
the community.*

Has stunted growth and shortened limbs that have
been noticeable since birth

*This describes a genetic growth disturbance, not
this syndrome.*

Has a noticeable limp when wearing shoes but not
in bare feet

*This describes an orthopedic problem or ill-fitting
shoes, not this syndrome.*

Has periods of "acting out" and misbehaving,
especially when there is company.

This sounds like a normal child.

ESSAY QUESTIONS

1. You are a nurse working in a shelter for battered women. They can live there with their children under the age of 14 for 2 months. What special considerations would you make to prevent abuse and neglect among the children while they live there? Identify three specific actions you would take.

2. You are discussing "shaken baby syndrome" with a family during a home visit at which you are teaching parenting skills. Describe how you would demonstrate how this occurs so that the family would not fear playing with their 6-month-old infant.

INDIVIDUAL OR GROUP PROJECTS

1. Have the students explore all services for battered women in the community. Compile a listing of the services with identifying data, including location, telephone numbers, services, and any other information useful to professionals and clients. Put this together in a booklet form and distribute to community health nurses, other professionals, and clients who might benefit from this information.

2. Have a group of students create a hand puppet play for preschool-aged children focusing on personal safety, good touch–bad touch, reporting inappropriate touching to a parent, and so on. Suggest that the students offer to present the play at preschools in your community.

Aggregates With Developmental Needs

CHAPTER 26

Maternal, Prenatal, and Newborn Populations

LEARNING OBJECTIVES

Upon mastery of this chapter, you should be able to:

- Discuss the global view of maternal and infant health.

- Identify the *Healthy People 2010* goals established for the maternal-infant population.

- Discuss major risk factors and special complications for childbearing families.

- Describe the important considerations in designing effective health promotion programs to fit the needs of diverse maternal-infant populations.

- List several features of a typical health promotion program for maternal-infant populations.

- Identify six methods of delivering services to maternal-infant populations.

- Describe various roles of a community health nurse in serving the maternal-infant population.

KEY TERMS

Developmental disability	Passive smoking
Drug dependent	Self-help groups
Drug exposed	Smokeless tobacco
Fetal alcohol effects	products
Fetal alcohol syndrome	Sudden infant death
Gestational diabetes mellitus	syndrome (SIDS)
Low birth weight	Very low birth weight

■ Teaching Strategies

CLASSROOM TEACHING STRATEGIES

1. Supply the class with the vital statistics on maternal and infant health, morbidity, and mortality for your city, county, and/or state, and have the students compare and contrast these statistics with the national statistics provided in Table 26-1 on page 515. Are the local statistics moving toward the 2010 goals in the objectives? If they are or are not, why or why not?

2. Hold a brainstorming session (Chapter 8) to generate a list of factors contributing to infant mortality and low-birth-weight infants in your community. From this list, have the class develop a community program to address these factors.

CLINICAL LABORATORY TEACHING STRATEGIES

1. Have the students prepare a teaching plan on a topic related to antepartum or postpartum nursing care. The plan should include objectives, topic content, teacher-learner activities including audio-visual materials and/or handouts, method of teaching, and method of evaluation. Provide the students with an opportunity to present their class to a group of pregnant or postpartum women and their families. Refer to Chapter 9 for teaching strategies, if this content has not been covered previously.

2. Have students locate a self-help group working with a maternal and infant population and attend a meeting. The students should return to the clinical laboratory group and be prepared to present the goals and accomplishments of the group to their peers. Do this early in the clinical laboratory experience so that the students will have information about support groups to share with clients during the span of the course.

ACTIVITIES TO PROMOTE CRITICAL THINKING IN THE CLASSROOM

1. Answer the questions in this activity in class. This would be especially important if the students will be working with the maternal-infant population in their clinical laboratory experience in community health nursing. Suggest that a small group of students gather this information as a small group project.

2. Answer the questions in this activity in class about halfway through the term, after the students have had several weeks in their clinical laboratory setting. Have a health department nursing supervisor speak to the class about the special maternal-infant programs the agency provides and what groups are especially targeted.

3. Discuss lifestyle-related factors that affect pregnant women and infants in your community. Draw from the clinical laboratory experiences of the students for specific case examples. What type of program is needed by this population that is not provided by the community at this time?

4. Use the case study in this activity with the class and have them participate in the exercise posed at the end of the scenario. Have the students in small enough groups of six to eight so that the group members can contribute to the planning designed to meet Sonia's needs.

5. Conduct this activity in class using the latest statistics available from the Internet (the students could find this information and bring it to class). Facilitate a discussion using the questions in this activity.

■ Evaluation Strategies

MULTIPLE-CHOICE QUESTIONS

1. In the United States the infant mortality rate for 1998 was:

   Higher than those of 24 other industrialized nations
   Even though U.S. infant mortality rates have improved, they remain higher than those in 24 other industrialized nations.

   Lower than those in Japan, France, and Italy
   The U.S.'s rates are higher than those in these three countries and 21 others.

   Four times higher among African-American than white mothers
   Infant mortality is twice as high among African-American women.

   Higher than decades earlier
   The rate was 7.2 per 1000 in 1998 compared to 20.0 in 1970. Our rates have improved, but not quickly enough or low enough.

2. Ineffective or failed community health care projects are often the result of:

   Incomplete assessment and lack of involvement of targeted populations
   Numerous projects have either failed or been ineffective because the targeted populations were assessed incompletely or not involved in the planning process.

   Designing a plan to meet specific identified needs
   This should help a project succeed and is not related to ineffective or failed projects.

   Failure to use a predetermined, generalized plan for all those served
   Such a plan will fail because it is not individualized for the target population.

   Identifying the developmental stage of the population being served
   This is an important part of the assessment, and projects do not fail because the developmental stage of the participants was identified.

3. Alcohol consumption during pregnancy has been *most* associated with infant:

   Intellectual impairment
   The health of infants can be dramatically affected by maternal consumption of alcohol. The pregnancy itself can be threatened. However, the most devastating consequence of alcohol consumption during pregnancy is FAE or FAS, both of which compromise the intellectual functioning of the infant or child.

   Low birth weight
   When pregnancy is threatened by alcohol consumption, a baby may have low birth weight. The most devastating long-term outcome is the impaired intellectual functioning of FAE or FAS.

   Respiratory distress
   This is not strongly associated with maternal alcohol consumption.

   Childhood cancers
   There is no association of childhood cancers with maternal alcohol consumption.

4. Smoking during pregnancy has been *most* associated with infant:

   Low birth weight
   The most common side effect on the fetus from maternal smoking during pregnancy is a lowered birth weight. Newborns weigh an average of 200 gm lower at birth in some studies. Other studies have shown that there is a greater incidence of stillbirths, spontaneous abortions, and perinatal mortality in pregnancies in which women smoke.

Genetic malformations
There is no association of genetic malformations with maternal smoking.

Developmental delays
There is no association of developmental delays with maternal smoking.

Feeding problems
There is no association of feeding problems with maternal smoking.

5. As part of teaching parenting to new parents, the community health nurse can demonstrate a method found to decrease the chance of sudden infant death syndrome (SIDS) when he or she:

Places infants on their backs as the preferred sleeping position
This is the recommended sleeping position for infants who cannot yet roll over. The Healthy People 2010 *target is to have 70% of infants put to sleep on their backs; the rate was 35% in 1996.*

Feeds infants while they are seated in an upright position
This is a good position to prevent infant choking— it will not prevent SIDS.

Never puts a baby down and props a bottle to feed the infant
This is a good recommendation to prevent choking, ear infections, and "bottle mouth" dental caries—it will not prevent SIDS.

Limits the time the infant spends in a mechanical swing
This is a good recommendation if an infant spends too much time in a swing—it will not prevent SIDS.

ESSAY QUESTIONS

1. Reflect on the pregnant women you have provided care to in the nursing program thus far. What high-risk behaviors (discussed in this chapter) did you observe in your clients? Did you discuss the behaviors with the clients? Did they change their high-risk behavior? What would you do differently now that you are taking community health nursing?

2. Reflect on the pregnancy of a person you know personally. What behaviors did she display that may be considered high-risk? Did you discuss the behavior(s) with her? Did any of her behaviors change because of you talking with her or as her pregnancy progressed? How different (culturally, socioeconomically, age) are the people you know personally from the pregnant clients you have cared for? Do these differences account for the differences in behaviors, if there were any?

INDIVIDUAL OR GROUP PROJECTS

1. Arrange for a group of students to visit the local, regional, or country health department or other community agency providing maternal-infant services and to meet with the director of those services. Questions that the students could ask the director might include the following:

   a. How many clients do they serve?

   b. What are the demographic and socioeconomic profiles of the clients?

   c. How do the clients qualify for prenatal care?

   d. What are the primary health concerns of women attending the clinic?

   e. What are the infant outcomes for women seen for prenatal care?

   Complete the project with a report to the entire class on the findings.

2. Arrange opportunities for students to teach a class or a series of classes on maternal and infant care (see Chapter 9 on teaching strategies). There are many community sites where maternal and infant populations gather, including clinics, WIC programs, childbirth education classes, nurse-midwives' offices, high schools, and nurse practitioner or physician offices.

CHAPTER 27

Promoting and Protecting the Health of Infant, Toddler, and Preschool Populations

LEARNING OBJECTIVES

Upon mastery of this chapter, you should be able to:

- Identify the changing demographics found in the infant, toddler, and preschool populations.

- Identify major health problems and concerns for infant, toddler, and preschool populations globally and in the United States.

- Describe a variety of programs that promote and protect health and prevent illness and injury of infant, toddler, and preschool populations.

- State the recommended immunization schedule for infants and children, and give the rationale for the timing of each immunization.

- Give examples of methods the community health nurse might use in working with infants, toddlers, and preschool populations to help promote their health.

KEY TERMS

Developmental disability
Drug dependent
Drug exposed
Fetal alcohol effects
Fetal alcohol syndrome
Gestational diabetes mellitus
Low birth weight

Passive smoking
Self-help groups
Smokeless tobacco
  products
Sudden infant death
  syndrome (SIDS)
Very low birth weight

∎ Teaching Strategies

CLASSROOM TEACHING STRATEGIES

1. Obtain vital statistics on infants and children from birth to age 5 for your community and state. Compare the mortality and morbidity rates against the goals in *Healthy People 2010*. Determine how close your local community and state comes to meeting these national health objectives, both at the baseline and the target rates.

2. Assess students for their willingness to share personal information about themselves, their siblings, and their own children. If they are receptive, discuss the group's personal expriences with childhood mortality and morbidity. How does the distribution compare with the morbidity and mortality causes highlighted in Chapter 27? Discuss differences and contemplate why there are differences.

CLINICAL LABORATORY TEACHING STRATEGIES

1. Have the students spend an observational/participatory day with a local preschool program. Compare and contrast practiced health behaviors: toilet facilities, handwashing practices of the children and staff, physical examination and immunization requirements before enrollment, quality and quantity of meals and snacks (do the children eat all the food?), napping and resting requirements, and so on. Discuss the differences during a clinical conference.

2. Have students plan and present a health promotion program for preschool children in a day-care setting or a Head Start program.

ACTIVITIES TO PROMOTE CRITICAL THINKING IN THE CLASSROOM

1. Have the students participate in this activity as a group in class. Select one of the leading causes of death among the infant-preschool population, such as accidents, and discuss a community-wide intervention that could be initiated to prevent these deaths.

2. Discuss with the students a possible health promotion program they could initiate and carry out in a day-care center during the term. If feasible, conduct this as part of the clinical laboratory experience.

3. Facilitate a general discussion on environmental hazards and how young children are especially at risk for them. What can a community health nurse do at the primary level of prevention to eliminate these hazards?

4. Discuss some of the lifestyle-related "nusisance" diseases (head lice, pubic lice, scabies, etc.) the students have encountered during their clinical laboratory experiences. How do you feel about caring for people with these diseases? If these same diseases appeared in the student's own family members, would they fell differently? What is the role of the community health nurse in relation to eradicating, eliminating, or controlling these diseases?

5. Include this activity in the classroom each term. This will facilitate building up ongoing statistics on how we, as a nation, are progressing toward meeting the *Healthy People 2010* goals with infants, toddlers, and preschool-aged children. As the years progress toward 2010, are we going to reach the goals? How does your local community measure up to the national statistics?

■ Evaluation Strategies

MULTIPLE-CHOICE QUESTIONS

1. On a global scale childhood mortality has been high. Fortunately, by 1995 it had declined to:

   Less than 1 in 10 children
   This was the global statistic for 1995.

   Twenty percent of children under age 5
   This was the global statistic for 1955.

   Less than 4 children per 100
   This is the expected number by 2025.

   One child per 100
   This would be a very ambitious statistic and currently is not predicted.

2. Infant mortality rates are considered an indicator of the general health status of a particular population. In the United States the mortality statistic in 2000 was:

   7.2 deaths per 1,000 live births
   This is the baseline statistic in Healthy People 2010. *Our 2010 target is 4.5.*

   99.9 deaths per 1,000 live births
   This is the statistic for 1915, when infant mortality rates were first recorded.

   47.0 deaths per 1,000 live births
   This is the statistic for 1940.

   2.6 deaths per 1,000 live births.
   This is the 1999 statistic for Iceland—well below our target of 4.5 for 2010.

3. The major cause of death in the birth-to-4-year-old population is:

   Unintentional injuries
   These cause most of the deaths for the birth-to-4-year old population—motor vehicle crashes, falls, drownings, fires, and burns.

   Pneumonia
   This is not a major cause of death in this population.

   Poverty
   Poverty contributes to many cases of morbidity and mortality but is not a cause of death in and of itself.

   Heart disease
   Heart disease is the fourth leading cause of death in this population.

4. Signs and symptoms of a young child with ADD include:

   Daydreaming and a lack of follow through
   The child with ADD displays signs and symptoms of a quieter nature than the child with ADHD. Symptoms such as not listening, losing things, and not paying attention are common (see Table 27-1 on page 544 of the textbook).

   Fidgeting and squirming when sitting
   This is a symptom of ADHD.

   Talking excessively
   This is a symptom of ADHD.

   Difficulty playing quietly
   This is a symptom of ADHD.

5. What is the primary cause of nutritional problems among the infant, toddler, and preschool population?

   Over-feeding and inappropriate food choices
   Many parents over-feed infants and toddlers and allow preschool-aged children to make imappropriate food choices, which can lead to a lifetime of nutritional problems.

   Living in the culture of poverty
   Although 20% of very young children live in poverty, the poverty itself does not cause nutritional problems.

   Cultural food preferences
   Although there are major differences in food preferences and eating practices among different cultural groups, they do not account for nutritional problems.

Experiencing growth spurts

Growth spurts in young children often are marked by changes in appetite, but it is the quality of the food than can cause the nutritional problems rather than infrequent changes in the quantity.

6. The community health nurse's role in providing health services to young children involves organizing programs for prevention of illness and injury, promotion of good health practices, and protection of health. Which of the following interventions would be classified as a protection activity?

Case finding and reporting

Case finding and reporting of communicable diseases, child abuse, child neglect, and so on protects children; thus, they are protection activities.

Immunization program

This is considered a preventive health program.

Early childhood development program

This is considered a health promotion program.

Nutrition program

This is considered a health promotion program.

ESSAY QUESTIONS

1. In 200 words or less, complete the following thought and describe what you would do to fulfill the role:. "If I were a nurse serving a preschool program, I would…"

2. Identify what a community health nurse should do at the three levels of prevention for infant, toddler, and preschooler passenger safety in automobiles.

INDIVIDUAL OR GROUP PROJECTS

1. Have a small group of students plan an infant-preschool health and safety fair at a local shopping mall or large toy store. The students would need to meet with the mall or store manager, complete a needs assessment, and contact appropriate agencies to participate in the fair. This same activity can be planned by three or four groups at different sites, held on different days using the same health and safety agency participation.

2. Arrange for students interested in community health, with a focus on infants and young children, to spend additional time in health department "well-baby" clinics and day-care and preschool programs monitored by community health nurses. Community health clinical laboratory objectives can be met in these settings, and many nurses would welcome the opportunity to share their expertise.

CHAPTER 28

Promoting and Protecting the Health of School-Aged and Adolescent Populations

LEARNING OBJECTIVES

Upon mastery of this chapter, you should be able to:

- Identify major health problems and concerns for school-aged and adolescent populations in the United States.

- Describe types of programs and services that promote health and prevent illness and injury of school-aged and adolescent populations.

- State the recommended immunization schedule for school-aged children and give the rationale for the timing of each immunization.

- Describe the three main functions of school nursing practice (health services, health education, and improvement of the school environment).

- Evaluate the potential benefits of school-based health centers, and discuss possible parental or community objections.

■ Key Terms

Anorexia nervosa	Pediculosis
Attention deficit hyperactivity disorder (ADHD)	School nurse
	School nurse practitioner
Bulimia	School-based health
Learning disability	center (SBHC)

■ Teaching Strategies

CLASSROOM TEACHING STRATEGIES

1. Obtain vital statistics on school-age children and adolescents for your community and state. Compare the mortality and morbidity rates against the goals in *Healthy People 2010*. Determine how close your local community and state comes to meeting these national health objectives, both at the baseline and the target rates.

2. Assess students for their willingness to share personal information about themselves, their siblings, and their own children. If they are receptive, discuss the group's personal experiences with childhood and adolescent mortality and morbidity. How does the distribution compare with the morbidity and mortality causes highlighted in Chapter 28? Discuss differences and contemplate why there are differences.

3. Invite two school nurses from the community to speak to the students about their roles with children and adolescents. How are the roles different based on the age of the children? Does one nurse get more involved in "hands-on" care than the other? Why? What screening programs does each nurse conduct? Do they use volunteers when conducting screening programs? Why or why not?

CLINICAL LABORATORY TEACHING STRATEGIES

1. Have the students spend an observational/participatory day with local school nurses at the elementary and high school levels. Compare and contrast school nursing roles during a clinical laboratory conference.

2. Have the students plan and present a health promotion program or a health fair for elementary or high school children. Such an activity could take place in the cafeteria or gymnasium during lunch time, recess, study hall periods, or just before or after school.

ACTIVITIES TO PROMOTE CRITICAL THINKING IN THE CLASSROOM

1. Facilitate a general discussion on the feelings and attitudes of the class regarding the use of medications for ADD/ADHD. Invite any of the students who have personal experience using such drugs in their families (siblings or their own children) to contribute to the discussion.

2. Have the students participate in this activity as a group in class. Select one of the leading causes of death among the childhood-adolescent population, such as accidental trauma, and discuss a community-wide intervention that could be initiated to prevent these deaths.

3. Use this activity to generate a general class discussion on values and attitudes toward people with diseases that are sexually transmitted. If the students have any clinical laboratory experiences that illustrate this dilemma, ask them to share the examples.

4. Use this activity to generate a general class discussion on the problem of nutrition in the school-aged and adolescent populations. You could divide the class into three small groups and have them discuss different aspects of this problem: programs available to encourage healthier diets, other factors that contribute to poor nutritional habits, and how the community health nurse works with parents, schools, and students to improve physical activity and nurtition. After allowing 20 to 30 minutes for this activity, have the groups share their findings and suggestions.

5. At some time during the term have two or three students spend a day with a school nurse who operates a school-based health center (as part of their clinical laboratory experience) and ask them to share their observations with the class. Ask them to seek out the answers to the questions in this activity.

6. Discuss the students' experiences with head lice in the clinical laboratory experience. Use the questions in this activity to stimulate discussion.

■ Evaluation Strategies

MULTIPLE-CHOICE QUESTIONS

1. Children under the age of 18 have a variety of chronic diseases. The most common chronic disease is:

Hay fever (allergic rhinitis)
This ranks first by condition prevalence.

Dermatitis
This ranks fifth by condition prevalence.

Acne
This ranks seventh by condition prevalence.

Heart disease
This ranks ninth by condition prevalence.

2. The major cause of death in the 5- to 14-year-old population is:

Accidental trauma
This causes most of the deaths in the 5- to 14-year-old population, the majority of which are from motor vehicle crashes.

Pneumonia
This is not a major cause of death in this population.

Poverty
Poverty contributes to many cases of morbidity and mortality but is not a cause of death in and of itself.

Chronic illnesses
Chronic illnesses contribute to the high morbidity among school-age children, but most chronic illnesses—such as hay fever, sinusitis, asthma (which is increasing and becoming more severe in some communities with urban density and high levels of pollution), bronchitis, dermatitis, orthopedic impairments, acne, and so on—are not life threatening.

3. The most effective school-based approach to solve the problem of teenage suicide includes:

Suicide prevention programs and direct interventions
Programs and interventions by couselors and school nurses that are focused on determining adolescent suicide intentions are the most effective approaches.

Teachers assessing suicide risk among students
Teachers do not feel comfortable or prepared to assess suicide risk, and this alone will not prevent teen suicide.

Promoting stronger parental control of teens
Peer pressure is strong, and parent concerns are not as important to the teen. Teens are seeking independence, and stronger parental control is not an effective method of reducing teen suicide.

Punitive treatment of teens by the school administration
This approach is inappropriate for any school-age child or teen behavior.

4. Violence among school-age children and adolescents is of concern to people in the United States. Statistics indicate that:

Homicide is the leading cause of death for African-American males 15 to 24 years old
Unfortunately, this is true, with this large minority group losing many young men due to violence.

Teen females commit suicide more frequently than
teen males
*They attempt suicide more, but male teens are more
successful; thus, their rates are higher.*

Homicide is the fifth highest cause of death for all
15- to 24-year-olds.
*Homicide is the second highest cause of death in
this age group.*

20% of all adolescent deaths are related to violence
The actual percentage is higher—40%.

5. In the 5 years between 1991 and 1996, teen birth
rates:

Declined in all ethnic groups and all states by 12%
*This is true. Teens are getting the message that teen
pregnancy can and should be avoided.*

Rose 24% from previous years
*This 24% rise occurred in the 5 years between 1986
and 1991.*

Continued to rise by 10% per decade, which it has
for 3 decades
*Teen pregnancy rose by 24% from 1986 to 1991
but decreased by 12% from 1991 to 1996.*

Doubled, placing public health officials on alert
*Public health care practitioners have always been
concerned (versus on alert) with the effects of
teenage pregnancy, but the rates have decreased
by 12%, not doubled.*

5. The specialty within community health nursing of
school nursing has its roots in:

The work of Lillian Wald in New York City in the
early 1900s
*Lillian Wald sent one of her nurses from the Henry
Stret Settlement to four schools in New York
City to decrease absenteeism, which was done
very successfully. This practice spread and the
school nurse movement began.*

England through the work of Florence Nightingale
*The school nurse movement began in the United
States through the work of Lillian Wald.*

Occupational health nursing in which nurses visited
the children of workers
*These movements occurred separately but at about
the same time in the early 1900s. Occupational
health nurses did not see children in schools.*

Schools where teachers were taught how to provide
nursing care to the children
*Lillian Wald sent one of her nurses from the Henry
Stret Settlement to four schools in New York
City to decrease absenteeism. It did not begin
with teachers providing nursing care.*

6. One of the three main functions of school nursing
practice is the promotion of a healthy school
environment. This includes which of the following?

The proper operation and maintenance of the
school buildings and grounds
*This is part of maintaining a healthy school
environment.*

Planned and incidental teaching of health concepts
*This is another function of school nursing
practice—health education.*

Curriculum development
*This is another function of school nursing
practice—health education.*

Vision, hearing, and scoliosis screening programs
*This is another function of school nursing
practice—health services.*

ESSAY QUESTIONS

1. In 200 words or less, complete the following
thought and describe what you would do to fulfill
the role. "If I were a school nurse I would..."

2. Identify the three levels of prevention for teenage
suicide.

INDIVIDUAL OR GROUP PROJECTS

1. Have a small group of students plan a health and
safety fair at a local school. The students would
need to meet with school officials, complete a needs
assessment, contact appropriate agencies to
participate in the fair, and plan the day and
location of the event. This same activity can be
planned by three or four groups at schools with
different age children (elementary, middle/junior
high school, and high school).

2. Arrange for students interested in school nursing to
spend some of their clinical laboratory hours with a
school nurse and have sufficient involvement to
participate in all aspects of the school nursing role.
Community health clinical laboratory objectives
can be met in this setting, and many school nurses
would welcome the opportunity to share their
expertise.

CHAPTER 29

Promoting and Protecting the Health of Adults and the Working Population

LEARNING OBJECTIVES

Upon mastery of this chapter, you should be able to:

- Identify key national and global demographic characteristics of adult men and women.

- Provide a health profile of adult men and women in the United States.

- Identify potential physical, chemical, biologic, ergonomic, and psychosocial stressors in a variety of work environments.

- Describe the history of state and federal legislation relative to occupational health.

- Discuss a variety of health problems related to occupation, including disorders related to ergonomics and workplace violence.

- Compare and contrast three main types of occupational health programs.

- Describe the role of the occupational health nurse and other members of the occupational health team in protecting and promoting workers' health and safety.

KEY TERMS

Adult	Occupational disease
Disabling injury	Occupational health
Employee assistance program	Occupational health nurse
Ergonomics	Unintentional injury
Life expectancy	Unsafe condition

■ Teaching Strategies

CLASSROOM TEACHING STRATEGIES

1. Have students share known occupational illnesses/injuries among their own family members. Do they relate more to health problems acquired in workers 20, 30, or 40 years ago than those younger family members working now? What makes the difference in the numbers and types of illnesses or injuries?

2. Invite an occupational health nurse to speak to the class about her or his role in business or industry.

CLINICAL LABORATORY TEACHING STRATEGIES

1. Suggest that students spend an observational day with an occupational health nurse to observe workers' health programs and the nurse's role in those programs.

2. Tour a large manufacturing plant with an occupational health nurse and have the clinical laboratory students identify potential and actual safety hazards, protective devices used, and health and safety programs for the employees. Discuss the group's observations during a clinical laboratory conference.

ACTIVITIES TO PROMOTE CRITICAL THINKING IN THE CLASSROOM

1. Peruse local newspapers for acts of violence in the workplace. Bring the articles to class and read them to the students. Have them identify how the violence might have been prevented.

2. Create a hypothetical company or use a company in your town that currently does not have a weight-control program. Have the students go through the steps to starting such a program for this company. As another approach, have the students work in small groups of six to eight and let them identify a hypothetical company, select a specific health promotion program, and then identify steps needed to implement the program. Have the students share their programs, and let the other groups critique the plans.

3. Discuss the potential and actual health-related risks associated with community health nursing. As a class, discuss ways to prevent or reduce these risks using the primary level of prevention.

4. Suggest that the students assess their clinical laboratory site(s) for health-related risks. Share them with the class. If appropriate, share the findings with nursing administration in the agency(ies).

■ Evaluation Strategies

MULTIPLE-CHOICE QUESTIONS

1. Every workplace has physical, chemical, biological, ergonomic, and psychosocial factors that affect health. Examples of ergonomic factors related to the worksite are things such as:

   Workplace design, tools, tasks, and equipment
   Ergonomic factors include the potential physiological and psychological stessors on the worker created by space allotments, tools, and physical positions workers must assume.

   Workplace temperature, light, noise, or vibration
   These are examples of physical factors in the workplace.

   Solvents, mists, vapors, or dusts in the workplace
   These are examples of chemical and biological factors in the workplace.

   Fatigue, anger, boredom, energy, and challenge on the job
   These are examples of psychosocial factors in the workplace.

2. Community health nurses need to be aware that the category of employees most exposed to bacteria, fungi, viruses, and molds includes:

   Agricultural workers
   Agricultural workers are potentially exposed to all of these bological factors, in addition to other ergonomic, physical, and chemical factors.

   Auto manufacturers
   The factors indicated do not usually affect auto manufacturers. They are exposed to ergonomic and physical factors more frequently.

   Painters
   The factors indicated do not usually affect painters. They are exposed to ergonomic and chemical factors more frequently.

   Photographers
   The factors indicated do not usually affect photographers. They are exposed to ergonomic and chemical factors more frequently.

3. Today's workers are protected by such significant legislation as the Workman's Compensation Act of 1910 and the Occupational Safety and Health Act (OSHA) of 1970. Which of the following is one aspect of the latter?

   Protects workers against injury and illness resulting from hazardous working conditions
   OSHA assures safe and healthful working conditions for men and women through development and enforcement of regulations and standards, maintenance of safety and health statistics, and worker safety education.

   Provides black lung benefits to aged and disabled coal miners
   These benefits were a part of the Federal Coal Mine Health and Safety Act of 1967.

   Provides injured workers with medical and rehabilitative care
   These benefits were first enacted as part of the Workman's Compensation Act of 1910.

   Protects workers by providing state and federal unemployment insurance
   These benefits are part of the Social Security Act of 1935.

4. Work-related illnesses and injuries cause more than 56,000 deaths annually. Some health-related problems present a particular concern to community health nurses and other health care workers because:

   For many illnesses there is a lag time between exposure, onset, and clinical evidence.
   A condition such as silicosis takes 15 years to develop. Some cases of mesothelioma (asbestos lung) may not become apparent for 25 years. Such illnesses and premature deaths are often difficult to trace back to a particular work environment.

   Industries are reluctant to report worker injuries.
   Industries must comply with OSHA record-keeping regulations. It would be difficult to hide worker injuries. Workers have unions and other mechanisms for employees to share their concerns about safety in the work setting.

   Methods have not been developed to enable occupational health researchers to make predictions.
   Research methods have been developed and researchers can make predictions. It is because of research that companies are striving to eliminate hazards in the work environment.

Workers hesitate to report safety concerns because of fear of losing their jobs.

In small work settings that escape the protection of OSHA, this may be a problem; however, in most work settings reporting safety concerns is expected and often rewarded, with departments listing "injury free" days and contests for the safest departments.

5. The Americans with Disabilities Act of 1990 was passed to:

Prevent discrimination against qualified workers with disabilities

This act has many facets. One aspect is to prevent discrimination against qualified workers.

Ensure that substances do not present an unreasonable health risk to workers

This is a part of the Toxic Substances Control Act of 1976.

Notify employees that there are hazards in the workplace that may cause disabilities

This is a part of the Hazard Communication Act of 1986.

Require employers to carry employee insurance

This is a part of the Workman's Compensation Act of 1910.

ESSAY QUESTIONS

1. Select one of the five (physical, chemical, biologic, ergonomic, or psychosocial) stressors that affect you in your work. List the aspects of that stressor that could affect your health, and identify what you can do about them to change the situation.

2. Occupational health nurses are usually not employed by small companies; however, if you had a company with 50 employees and could "contract" for the services of an occupational health nurse 8 hours a week, what would you have the nurse focus on in the time allowed? Your company produces gourmet ice cream and operates 16 hours a day, 6 days a week.

INDIVIDUAL OR GROUP PROJECTS

1. Have a group of students complete an assessment on a small local company (with the company's cooperation) as an external review service. Determine the positive and negative aspects of the company's health and safety program. Share the results with the company occupational health nurse or safety director and classmates, and make suggestions for safety improvements, if necessary.

2. If students are currently employed in a health care setting, suggest that they assess their hospital unit, agency, or service for adequacy of health and safety standards. If hazards exist, the student should share the information with a supervisor. The student should write a report including the area's strengths and weaknesses.

CHAPTER 30

Promoting and Protecting the Health of the Older Adult Population

LEARNING OBJECTIVES

Upon mastery of this chapter, you should be able to:

- Describe the global and national health status of older adults.

- Identify and refute at least four common misconceptions about older adults.

- Describe characteristics of healthy older adults.

- Provide an example of primary, secondary, and tertiary prevention practices among the older population.

- Discuss four primary criteria for effective programs for older adults.

- Describe various living arrangements and care options for older adults.

- Describe the future of an aging America and the role of the community health nurse.

KEY TERMS

Ageism	Gerontology
Alzheimer's disease	Group home
Assisted living	Hearty elderly
Baby boomers	Hospice care
Board and care homes	Intermediate care
Case management	Long-term care
Confidant	Osteoporosis
Continuing care center	Personal care homes
Custodial care	Respite care
Elite-old	Senility
Frail elderly	Skilled nursing facility
Geriatrics	

■ Teaching Strategies

CLASSROOM TEACHING STRATEGIES

1. Have students describe their perceptions of elderly persons. They can do this by writing poems or short essays. Simply give them the title of "Older People" as an assignment. Have the poems and short stories copied and distributed to each student

(with permission of the students), and discuss the feelings and perceptions described in the poems.

2. Invite elderly members of the community (a retired community health nurse, a centenarian who lives in the community, etc.) to speak to the class. Discuss the following topics and how many of these have changed since they were young:

    a. Lifestyle changes related to aging

    b. Health needs

    c. Social support systems

    d. Hobbies and recreational activities

    e. Transportation changes/problems, if any

    f. Perceptions about how others feel about aging and how they feel about their own aging (add additional topics relevant to your community)

CLINICAL LABORATORY TEACHING STRATEGIES

1. Have students carry out the following activities:

    a. Complete a community assessment to gather data on the elderly population and prioritize the identified needs.

    b. Speak to a member of the local police force regarding safety issues of seniors within the community.

    c. Speak to a representative of the department of Health and Human Services or Area Agency on Aging regarding elder abuse, economic security, and alternatives to institutional care.

2. Have students use data obtained from the vital statistics of a predetermined census tract and other community sources to determine the following information:

    a. The number of elderly people in the community

    b. Where the elderly live (location, type of housing)

    c. The needs of the following age groups in areas such as health, recreation, transportation, and so on: 65 to 74 years old, 75 to 84, 85 and older

ACTIVITIES TO PROMOTE CRITICAL THINKING IN THE CLASSROOM

1. Complete this activity in class. Ask for students to describe an older adult (over 65, 75, or 85—decide on a specific age) whom everyone knows—a retired faculty member, a local business person or politician, and so on. Describe her or his characteristics. How many of these characteristics fit the students' picture of a senior citizen? Do the characteristics change if you select someone over 65 versus over 85?

2. Do any students make home visits to a client or have a family member who resembles Minnie Blackstone? If so, discuss how a community health nurse could interact with her to maintain and promote her health.

3. If the students visit a group of seniors during their clinical laboratory experience, discuss what programs, services, and activities the students are involved in, have started, or are planning to conduct as part of their work with these elders. What additional services might be provided in the future by other students?

4. As a class, discuss the process of doing a needs assessment in relation to potential program planning for elders in the community. Define the steps needed to be taken.

5. After small groups of students have visited a continuing care center, an assisted living center, or secure senior housing, discuss which types of housing options they would consider for themselves—why or why not?

6. Ask the students to share their Internet findings about innovative programs for elders. Ask them to describe them to the class. Would any of these programs work in your community? If the group feels there is a need for such a service, suggest that a task force of students approach the appropriate agency and share the program or services with them.

▪ Evaluation Strategies

MULTIPLE-CHOICE QUESTIONS

1. One important task that nurses should perform in working with an elderly population in the community is:

   Developing case management programs to channel clients to appropriate services
   Services for the elderly should be proactive. Nurses should design interventions that maximize nursing resources and provide the greatest benefit to elderly clients.

   Placing the elderly in skilled nursing facilities so they can have the best care available
   Skilled nursing facilities are for people with skilled needs, not for older adults managing chronic diseases independently. One's own home is most often the best place for elders and where they want to be.

   Raising funds to support the needs of the elderly in the community
   This is not something that is always needed or possible for a community health nurse to become involved in. Nurses can identify the needs for additional funding, advocate for more funding, and facilitate a community group's efforts to raise funds. This is how a nurse can best serve the elderly and support their needs rather than by actually raising the funds.

   Emphasizing tertiary prevention at this stage in the lives of the elderly
   Prevention should be proactive and focus on primary prevention regardless of the client's age.

2. Chronic diseases are common among older adults. Select the statement that most accurately reflects older adults and chronic diseases.

   Postural hypotension can be related to falls in elders.
   Older adults need to have sufficient cerebral circulation to avoid dizziness. Dizziness can lead to falling. A normal to high-normal blood pressure for the elder should be maintained.

   Forty percent of older adults are diagnosed with diabetes.
   In 1999 it was estimated that 18.4% of people over 65 have diabetes.

   Weight-bearing exercises are related to increased cases of osteoporosis.
   Weight-bearing exercises are a way to prevent osteoporosis at the primary level.

Older white men have the highest rates of hypertension among the major racial groups in the U.S.

Older African-American men have the highest rates of hypertension.

3. The study of all aspects of the aging process is included in:

Gerontology

Gerontology includes the economic, social, clinical, and psychological aspects of older adults and society.

Geriatrics

This is the medical specialty that deals with the physiology of aging and with the diagnosis and treatment of diseases affecting the aged.

Case management

This is the coordinated system of care provided to people with illnesses of all ages.

Gastrology

This is the study of the function and diseases of the stomach.

4. Community health nurses work in continuing care centers. What is unique about these centers is that they:

Provide a variety of housing and care options that elders need as they age

They are comprehensive centers and have become the last place an older adult needs to live, meeting independent to dependent needs, including skilled nursing and Alzheimer's disease services (see Display 30-9 on page 619).

Accept only clients needing skilled nursing services

They accept residents at all stages of need, from totally independent living to assisted living to skilled nursing care. In some settings, residents cannot enter the residence at the skilled nursing level. These beds are filled by residents with increasing needs as they move from independent living, to assisted living, to skilled nursing care.

Are similar to board and care homes

These small, 6- to 12-bed "homes" provide, at most, assisted and hospice services. They do not meet all the potential skilled needs of an older adult.

Are respite centers for family members of older adults

Friends and family can visit, and in independent and assisted living areas family and friends can spend the night. They are not designed for family members but as permanent residences for elders.

5. A specific goal for older adults in *Healthy People 2010* includes:

A reduction to 20% of older adults 65 to 74 years old who have lost all of their teeth

This is the Healthy People 2010 goal. There was a baseline of 26% in 1997.

Reduce the suicide rate for older white men to 50.0 per 100,000

We surpassed the Healthy People 2000 target of 38.9 3 years early with 35.5 per 100,000. Suicide continues to be of concern in the Healthy People 2010 objectives but is well below 50.0 per 100,000.

Reduce elders' fears of crime to 50% of those people over 65

This is not a goal within the Healthy People 2010 document. However, 24% of elders consider the fear of crime a major concern.

Extending years to the expected life-span

Healthy People 2010 is more specific. There is no value in extending years of life if the quality of life is poor. Healthy People 2010's goal is to extend the healthy years of life.

ESSAY QUESTIONS

1. Using the prase, "When I am 85 years old, I will...," complete your thoughts in as much detail as possible.

2. Describe briefly an older adult you know. Develop a health promotion plan for him or her based on strategies for successful aging proposed by Dr. Walter Bortz (1996) in his book, *Dare to be 100.*

INDIVIDUAL OR GROUP PROJECTS

1. Interview a group of seniors at a senior center as part of a needs assessment for the agency. What wants and needs do the participants identify? Which ones can a community health nurse help to meet?

2. Using the information gathered in individual or group project 1, plan several programs to meet the needs and wants of the attendees at the senior center.

UNIT VII

Vulnerable Aggregates

CHAPTER 31

Rural Clients

LEARNING OBJECTIVES

Upon mastery of this chapter, you should be able to:

- Define the term rural.

- Discuss population characteristics of rural residents.

- Identify at-risk populations in rural communities.

- Describe five barriers to health care access for rural clients.

- Relate the broad objectives of *Healthy People 2010* to the concept of "social justice" in rural communities.

- Discuss activities to assist in the orientation of a new community health nurse to a rural community.

- Compare and contrast the "circle of continuity of care" and the "circle of family and community support" themes apparent in rural communities.

- Discuss the challenges and opportunities related to rural community health nursing practice.

KEY TERMS

Circle of continuity of care
Circle of family and
    community support
Frontier area
Health professional
    shortage area (HPSA)
Key informant

Metropolitan
Nonmetropolitan
Out-migration
Rural
Telehealth
Urban area (UA)

■ Teaching Strategies

CLASSROOM TEACHING STRATEGIES

1. Discuss the differences in completing a community assessment in rural areas versus urban areas. Where would community health nurses go for assessment data? Does the value of key community leaders' information change? Would long-term community members' memories be important to tap into?

2. Discuss who are the rural populations at risk. How can a community health nurse work with these groups effectively in rural communities? Are there specific barriers that must be overcome?

CLINICAL LABORATORY TEACHING STRATEGIES

1. If possible, seek out rural clinical laboratory experiences for the students. They may be easy to find and possible on a full-time basis during the course if you are located in a rural part of your state. If you are located in an urban setting, find an opportunity for the students to observe or provide services in a rural community health nursing setting one or two times during the term. Such possibilities may include working in a migrant work camp clinic, on an Indian reservation or Rancheria, or in a rural satellite clinic.

2. Perhaps you have an opportunity to have students observe a home health nurse who works with rural clients, a school nurse who works in a rural school, or a midwife who serves rural perinatal families. If so, ask the students to share their observational experience with the clinical laboratory students during a clinical conference. How do the roles of these nurses compare and contrast with nurses working in the same roles in urban or suburban settings?

ACTIVITIES TO PROMOTE CRITICAL THINKING IN THE CLASSROOM

1. Facilitate a short discussion among the students, focusing on those who grew up in rural communities. Determine what they consider to be their best experiences growing up. Compare these experiences with those students who grew up in urban or suburban areas.

2. After the students complete this assignment, discuss the differences between the rural and urban assessments among the whole class.

3. Use the scenario that the students are community health nurses in a rural community. Discuss their approaches to solving the problem of overuse of the emergency room for minor childhood illnesses by the rural community residents.

4. Suggest that the students share their findings from the Internet regarding rural job opportunities for community health nurses.

■ Evaluation Strategies

MULTIPLE-CHOICE QUESTIONS

1. According to various U.S. official definitons, the term "frontier area" is a community having:

   Fewer than six people per square mile
   This is the U.S. government's definition of "frontier area."

   A population density of fewer than 1,000 people per square mile
   This is the U.S. Bureau of the Census' definition of "rural."

   Counties without a city of 50,000 residents
   This is the U.S. Office of Management and Budget's definition of "non-metropolitan."

   Fewer than 2,500 urban population either adjacent to or not adjacent to a metropolitan area
   This is the U.S.D.A. Rural-Urban Continuum Codes definition of "completely rural."

2. As a way to describe rural clients as a whole, you could say that they are most typically:

   Older, white, with a lower income and less formal education
   Although people of all ages, races, income, and education levels live in rural America, the rural population as a whole is significantly older; more are Caucasian; fewer are college graduates and more are high school dropouts; and generally rural Americans have a lower income.

   Young minorities with a lower income and less formal education
   They are older and white with a lower income and less formal education.

   Wealthier, more highly educated, older white Americans
   Although some rural inhabitants are wealthy and highly educated, most are older, white, with a lower income and less formal education.

   A reflection of the population as a whole
   The rural population does not reflect the whole population. It is older, white, with a lower income and less formal education.

3. As an aggregate, rural elders are at special risk. This is related to:

   Their increased chronic diseases along with barriers to access to specialists
   Rural elders have the same increasing chronic diseases as all elders nationwide but have barriers to accessing needed specialists, as most physicians practice in urban or suburban areas.

   The overwhelmingly poor health of rural elders
   They have health problems at about the same rate as urban or sururban elders, with an additional barrier of access to health care.

   The increasing numbers of rural elderly seeking out alternative housing arrangements
   Rural elders stay at home and try to maintain independence longer than urban or suburban elders, who have more alternative housing choices.

   Their refusal to use the bevy of community services needed to maintain them at home
   Many of the community services required to maintain ill elders in their homes may not be available in rural communities.

4. Cardiovascular disease is the number one health problem in the United States. Among rural inhabitants it is a more significant problem. This is related to:

   Limited use of preventive interventions and ignoring early cardiovascular symptoms
   Because of access barriers in rural areas to quality health care facilities and less access to preventive health information, rural inhabitants have a higher incidence of cardiovascular disease and poorer outcomes once diagnosed.

   Eating a diet consisting of fresh farm foods that may be high in animal and vegetable fats
   Many rural inhabitants eat high-fat diets but do so in conjunction with lack of exercise and smoking. Farm families who are physically active and do not smoke are not hindered by eating fresh farm foods.

   Rural inhabitants not trusting medical practitioners and the health care delivery system
   The problem is lack of access, not trust. There are limited medical practitioners and less high-tech equipment available, which may affect outcomes for rural patients with cardiovascular emergencies.

   The high number of people moving to rural areas, which impacts the health care system
   Although urban and suburban areas are sprawling outward and taking over once existing farm land, the numbers of people actually moving to rural areas are not high. In addition, population shifts are not causing increased cases of cardiovascular disease or poor outcomes once diagnosed.

5. Rural community health nursing is different from community health nursing in urban and suburban areas. One of the differences noted is that rural community health nurses experience:

Closer ties to the community and less burnout than their urban counterpart

They know the resources in the community and are a part of it, and they have less burnout than urban community health nurses.

Burnout at greater rates because they are expected to be all things to all people

Although they may be expected to be all things to all people, they experience less burnout.

Being seen as just another worker and not a positive asset to the community

On the contrary, they are seen as positive assets to their community.

Clear definitions between social and professional roles

There is a blurring of social and professional roles for the rural community health nurse.

ESSAY QUESTIONS

1. Suggest that students write a short paper about their experiences growing up in urban, suburban, or rural areas. This kind of assignment would be graded as full credit for completing the assignment, or the grade is based on insight and other points you spell out in the instructions. Complete the following sentence: "What I learned most from growing up in a rural/suburban/urban area that will help me as a community health nurse is..."

2. Select one of the rural populations at risk discussed in the textbook (homeless families, perinatal families, the elderly, the mentally ill, Native Americans, or farm workers) and discuss a specific program you would promote to assist this population.

INDIVIDUAL OR GROUP PROJECTS

1. Select one of the rural populations at risk you have been working with in your clinical laboratory experience and, working in small groups, plan and implement a service or program you can complete during the term. Such activities as a health fair, flu-immunization clinic, or a bike-safety clinic might be welcomed. Where would you conduct your program? With whom would you collaborate to ensure a successful event?

2. If interested in rural nursing, compile a listing of rural job opportunities from a variety of sources such as the Internet, professional nursing journals, or local newspapers. If nearing the end of the nursing program, communicate with the hiring agency, visit the facility, or in some way begin to seriously explore job opportunities. Are there special funds for health care professionals that reimburse for college if you work in a rural area for a specified period of time? Use the Internet to explore the possibilities.

CHAPTER 32

Clients Living in Poverty

LEARNING OBJECTIVES

Upon mastery of this chapter, you should be able to:

- Identify common characteristics of people living in poverty.

- Analyze political and ethical dimensions of American poverty.

- Identify common health effects of poverty.

- Analyze causes of homelessness and the effect on health.

- Explain the forces determining global poverty and strategies for its elimination.

- Propose intervention strategies at the community, agency, and individual level.

- Assess your own attitude toward poverty and identify self-caring strategies when working with impoverished people.

KEY TERMS

Disenfranchised
Distributive justice
Feminization of poverty
Homelessness
Indigent
Marginalized

Poverty threshold
Social status
Social support
Temporary Aid to Needy
   Families (TANF)

■ Teaching Strategies

CLASSROOM TEACHING STRATEGIES

1. Use the Clinical Corner situation in this chapter as a classroom activity. Have the students work in small groups to answer the four discussion questions at the end of the exercise on page 655.

2. Ask the students to identify some of their current behaviors that might indicate that, as students, they are living in situational poverty. Do they live in housing they would not consider once they graduate and are employed? Are they currently not covered by health insurance and hoping they stay well? Do they buy "store brands," dented cans, or shop in discount grocery stores? Do they collect, recycle, and get money for aluminum cans, plastic, or newspapers? Discuss some of these behaviors as possible resources to share with clients, or suggest that the students pick up dollar-stretching ideas from their clients—making them the "experts."

CLINICAL LABORATORY TEACHING STRATEGIES

1. Discuss clients that the students are visiting in the clinical laboratory setting in relation to any acute or chronic illnesses they have. Are any related to the condition of poverty? How would the health of the clients be different if they were not living in poverty?

2. Discuss clients living in poverty to whom students provide services in the clinical laboratory setting. Are any of the families receiving Temporary Aid to Needy Families (TANF) from the state? What are their plans when they become ineligible for these funds (see pages 645–646)? Do the students have a role in anticipatory guidance in helping the family reach financial independence successfully?

ACTIVITIES TO PROMOTE CRITICAL THINKING IN THE CLASSROOM

1. Implement this activity as a class. Suggest that small groups of students compile the costs for a simple nutritional diet, housing for a family of four, basic clothing for a family of four, and other basic necessities such as transportation, utilities, and emergency funds. How does this cost compare with the most recent poverty threshold established by the government?

2. Ask the students to share, if they feel comfortable, their own experiences with poverty in their family. Is it something easy to talk about? Is it a family secret?

3. Ask the students to drive around their own neighborhood and look for pockets of poverty, as demonstrated by the condition of the housing and upkeep of the yards, streets in ill repair, reports and observations of drug dealing and increased crime, condition and number of automobiles, and so on. When they look objectively at their neighborhood, is there more poverty or low-income families living there than they initially thought? What do county statistics show regarding crime, income, density of housing, and so on in the community the students grew up in? Are they surprised by these findings?

4. Discuss the students' comparisons between impoverished communities and affluent communities and the resources available to each.

5. Initiate a discussion about the worth of human beings. Is an individual's worth measured by his or her education, employment, and material goods?

6. Initiate a discussion on the question, "How do the poor contribute to their poverty?" Are they responsible for it?

7. Use the two case scenarios described in Displays 32-1 and 32-2 and answer the questions as a class for both cases.

8. In the election year 2000, California had on its ballot an opportunity to assign non-violent drug users to medical treatment on first and second offenses instead of receiving a jail sentence. Other states may have this already, or it may appear on ballots in your state in the future. How do you feel about such changes in the law? Is drug use a crime or an illness or both? What do you feel is the best way to manage offenders?

9. Initiate a discussion focusing on the concept of whether basic shelter and food are rights or privileges. Ask students to defend and support the view they hold.

10. Ask the students to share their experiences and observations while sitting in a public health clinic or welfare agency. How were people treated? How would you feel if this was a clinic or social service agency you had to use? Compare this with how you are treated at your private health care provider's office.

11. Open this question up to the class for discussion. Do the students have negative stereotypes about poor people? What can each student do to change some of his or her attitudes if they are negative?

■ Evaluation Strategies

MULTIPLE-CHOICE QUESTIONS

1. The demographics of poverty include the following statistic:

   Most impoverished Americans are white.
   This is true, but the largest single group of Americans is white. Compared with their presence in the population, a disproportionate number of people of color are poor.

   Twenty-five percent of the U.S. population was poor in 1998.
   The actual number was 13% in 1998.

   The number of extremely poor people is decreasing.
   The number is increasing. In 1997, 14.6 million Americans were classified as extremely poor—those people trying to survive on less than half of the official poverty line.

   Thirty percent of the elderly live below the poverty line.
   The number is 10%, with 17% considered "near poor" with incomes less than 125% of the poverty line.

2. The lifestyle of people living in poverty is marked by the following trait:

   Cash is chronically short, with money being borrowed at inflated interest rates.
   Unemployment or being employed at low wages in unskilled work causes a chronic cash problem. The poor, with few assets, borrow money from lenders who charge high interest rates.

   Attitudes and behaviors include optimism and mainstream organizational involvement.
   Attitudes and behaviors usually include fatalism and marginal connection to mainstream organizations.

   The lifestyle includes future orientation and postponement of immediate gratification.
   The lifestyle includes present-day orientation and little postponement of immediate gratification.

   There is a belief in their ability to influence the course of their lives.
   Most do not believe that they can influence the course of their lives.

3. In 1996 the Aid to Families with Dependent Children (AFDC) program was restructured into Temporary Aid to Needy Families (TANF). The most significant change to the program is that:

   Family support has a 5-year lifetime limit and the recipient must find work within 2 years
   These are the basics of the TANF program, which dramatically revamps the AFDC program.

Financial support ends when the youngest child reaches age 5 and is in school full time

This is not a part of TANF. The heart of the TANF plan is that family support has a 5-year lifetime limit and the recipient needs to find work within 2 years.

Child care provisions for the recipients of TANF are required by federal law

There are no federal mandates to make child care provisions available, although it is known that such help enables families to escape poverty.

More people are eligible for Medicaid under the TANF reforms

Many people have lost Medicaid coverage and become uninsured as a result of the TANF reforms.

4. People living in poverty have increased morbidity and mortality. Which of the following situations, if they exist in poor communities, needs to be interrupted in order to improve conditions?

The breakdown of social bonds and lowered social trust

This contibutes to high morbidity and mortality rates and needs to be interrupted.

Living in high-trust neighborhoods where people share resources

This decribes a positive condition and, despite poverty, people are healthier; thus, it should be encouraged, not interrupted.

Decreasing smoking, physical inactivity, and overweight conditions

Persons with the least education and lowest income are the most likely to smoke, overeat, and be physically inactive. Any decrease in these activities should be promoted and continued, not interruped.

Becoming empowered to overcome the limitations poverty bestows on people

If a community becomes empowered, they can overcome the limitations of poverty and change their circumstances. This should be encouraged, not interrupted.

5. The eradication of global poverty is on the agenda for the United Nations. Which of the following actions is being proposed by the United Nations?

Fair trade policies that allow poor countries to enter the world market

This is one of the actions being proposed by the United Nations.

Promotion of strong authoritarian governments who represent the people

There must be support for governments to be accountable, open, and with active citizen participation.

Empowerment of men in communities

Empowerment of women is what is needed. Most women in underdeveloped countries are not empowered.

Suggesting that people in poor communities begin acting individually

There needs to be support for poor communities to organize and act collectively. An individual voice will not give the power and leadership a country needs.

ESSAY QUESTIONS

1. Consider some of the health effects of homelessness shared in this chapter. Select one and give examples of actions a community health nurse can take to prevent such an effect at the primary level of prevention.

2. One of the roles of a community health nurse in caring for aggregates living in poverty is strengthening the community. Using a community you have served during the term in the clinical laboratory experience, discuss actions you could take to strengthen it.

INDIVIDUAL OR GROUP PROJECTS

1. Select a classroom in an elementary school in a poor neighborhood. Work with the teacher to provide intensive health-promotion activities with the children during the school term as part of the nursing students' clinical laboratory experience. If the numbers of nursing students are sufficient, select more than one class, such as all the first grades in the school. This might be an activity that can be conducted each year, which would provide the school with ongoing health care information to the whole school population after a few years.

2. Develop an educational program on nutrition that is appropriate for a group of elders who live in poverty and attend a neighborhood senior center. Include in this program ways to stretch their food dollar, getting the best buys at grocery stores, buying in bulk and sharing with neighbors, taking advantage of surplus food programs available to seniors in some communities, and so on. Encourage the students to stretch their imaginations and to collaborate with a nutritionist or other community senior advocates to develop a useful program.

CHAPTER 33

Migrant Workers

LEARNING OBJECTIVES

Upon mastery of this chapter, you should be able to:

- Discuss the historical background of migrant workers and their demographics and patterns.

- Describe the migrant lifestyle.

- Explain how hazardous living and working conditions contribute to migrant workers' increased risk for health problems.

- Identify at least three health problems common to migrant workers and their families.

- Describe social issues resulting from the migrant lifestyle.

- Discuss barriers and challenges to migrant health care.

- Identify methods for effective health care delivery to migrant populations.

- Discuss goals and implications for effective health care delivery to migrant populations.

KEY TERMS

Camp health aide	Migrant farmworker
Crew leader	Migrant health program
Cultural brokering	Migrant streams
Cultural sensitivity	Outreach
Curanderas	Patterns of migration
Familialism	Personalismo
Homebase	Seasonal farmworker
Lay workers	Simpatica
Machismo	

■Teaching Strategies

CLASSROOM TEACHING STRATEGIES

1. Ask a community health nurse who serves a migrant work camp to speak to the class and discuss her or his role. Have the nurse speak about common health problems and health risks related to the type of farm work the workers are engaged in.

2. If possible, ask a migrant family to come to class and discuss their personal experience working at various farms. They may be more comfortable sharing their story as a part of a panel discussion or a seminar. Perhaps a nursing student knows the family, or they are part of an advocacy group for migrant workers, or are well known to the community health nurse who serves their camp.

CLINICAL LABORATORY TEACHING STRATEGIES

1. If possible, have students spend some of their clinical laboratory experience time with migrant populations. This can be done in a mobile clinic, at a migrant workers' camp, or in a Head Start or school program for migrant workers. If this is not possible for the class as a whole, have at least one or two students observe in one of the settings.

2. Provide educational programs for the children of migrant workers who attend school in communities you serve during your clinical laboratory experience. Consider the need to conduct them in Spanish or to use simple language that children who speak English as a second language can understand. Work with the school administration and individual classroom teachers to produce a useful program.

ACTIVITIES TO PROMOTE CRITICAL THINKING IN THE CLASSROOM

1. Use the quote from this activity, "Justice in the fields slips through the fingers like a handful of soil," and discuss what it means to each student.

2. Discuss the health-related topics mentioned in this activity and why these specific topics are appropriate for migrant populations.

3. Using the topics covered in this inventory, discuss how they contribute to stress in migrant families' lives.

4. Discuss your feelings about the government's decision to discontinue federal food stamps for hundreds of thousands of legal immigrants without plans for alternatives. Do you support this decision? Why or why not?

5. Facilitate a discussion on the nomadic lifestyle experienced by migrant workers. How do you think you would have fared if your family had been migrant workers? Would you be a nursing student now?

■ Evaluation Strategies

MULTIPLE-CHOICE QUESTIONS

1. Cesar Chavez is mentioned in this chapter as:

   Founder of the United Farm Workers who spent his life fighting for social justice
   Cesar Chavez founded the UFW, fought for social justice, and is an example of an outstanding migrant hero.

   A Mexican president who worked to keep people from crossing the border illegally
   This does not describe Cesar Chavez's work.

   A well-known actor who advocates for increasing the number of Latinos in Hollywood
   This does not describe Cesar Chavez's work.

   The senator who wrote the Children's Health Insurance Program (CHIP) bill
   This does not describe Cesar Chavez's work.

2. Migrant workers are composed of farm laborers who work in:

   Every state in the union and are often "invisible" members of society
   They work in all states. Their numbers are concentrated along the southern border of the country and the eastern and western states.

   Only the southern and western states that border Mexico
   This is a misconception. Migrant farm workers work all over the United States.

   Farms owned by foreign corporations, thus not coming under U.S. government laws.
   Migrant workers are employed by anyone who hires them and should follow all laws of the country, especially those of legal residency and health requirements.

   Farms in the migrant streams, avoiding other farms worked by nonmigrant workers
   Migrant farmers work on all farms. Some are along a path of agriculture in the United States called migrant streams or migrant patterns. However, migrant workers are employed by any farmer needing help with crop planting or harvesting.

3. The health statistics for migrant families are shocking and include:

   A life expectancy that is 66% the national average
   Life expectancy is 49, cutting one third off of the life of these workers.

   A hospitalization rate of migrant families that is 25% above the national average
   The hospitalization rate is 50% higher than the national average for the country as a whole.

   A death rate from communicable diseases that is 10 times higher than the national average
   The death rate from TB and other communicable diseases is 25 times higher than the national average.

   A 50% increase in migrant infant mortality rates
   Migrant infants experience a mortality rate that is 125% higher than the national average.

4. A community health nurse works to offer increased health care services to meet the needs of a local migrant population. Which of the following ideas will work well for this population?

   Providing a mobile van clinic that comes to the farms during the day
   This would help the greatest number of migrant family members, as most of the family members are working all day.

   Offering a clinic at the migrant camp during the day
   All family members work in the fields. Women work alongside the men. Children work if they are old enough, or they are in school. Babies and young children accompany the parents to the fields. Generally, there is no one at the migrant camp during the day.

   Asking local doctors to stay open until 6 PM in the evenings in the summer
   Migrant workers are in the fields until dark. In the summer that may be 9 PM; thus, a physician who stays open until 6 PM will not help.

   Offering school-based clinic sites for migrant farm families to use
   This conflicts with work hours, and transportation to the school would be another barrier.

5. The role of community health nurses in caring for migrant workers includes:

   Employing information tracking systems
   This is necessary due to the mobility of this population and the need for continuity of care.

   Maintaining existing services
   The nurse should improve the existing services.

   Using standard methods of health care delivery
   Nurses need to use unique methods of health care delivery to reach this population.

   Using professionals for community outreach
   This population is best reached by using lay personnel for community outreach.

ESSAY QUESTIONS

1. Provide the students with a case study of a migrant farm family, mention several early symptoms of beginning health problems they experience, and describe the type of work they do. Have the students develop a family visit plan to promote the health of this family.

2. Take the same case study and suggest that the students prepare a lesson plan for a 30-minute class on primary prevention of one of the types of health problems migrant families may experience because of the type of work they do. Examples include urinary tract infections (due to lack of toileting facilities in the fields) aggravated by bending, stooping, and squatting all day to work, or contact dermatitis from exposure to pesticides.

INDIVIDUAL OR GROUP PROJECTS

1. Develop a file of current articles on migrant health or migrant nursing and give it to the community health nursing staff in the agency where you have clinical laboratory experience as a resource for their work with migrant families. If your community has few migrant families, does it have a large immigrant population? If so, develop a similar file on working with families new to the United States and their specific health care needs.

2. Students sometimes become involved in gift giving at holiday times during the school year. Organizing the resources needed for these gifts takes teamwork, organization, knowledge of community resources, and volunteerism. As part of a special gift for a migrant family, a classroom of migrant children, or a migrant camp, solicit donations from local businesses or work together as a class to raise funds for special items. Items that may be useful include clothing store gift certificates or blankets for an individual family; a computer or art supplies for the classroom; or bedding, large bags of rice, or disposable diapers for migrant camp families.

CHAPTER 34

Clients With Mental Health Issues

LEARNING OBJECTIVES

Upon mastery of this chapter, you should be able to:

- Discuss the historical evolution of mental health care.

- Explain the obstacle of stigma in community mental health.

- Discuss the incidence and prevalence of mental illness in the U.S.

- Describe the risk factors affecting the mentally ill population.

- Discuss the needs of and treatment approaches for the mentally ill population.

- Identify and describe community mental health resources.

- Describe preventive interventions for the mentally ill population at each level of the public health prevention model.

- Define health promotion and discuss health-promoting interventions for community mental health.

- Describe six aspects of the nurse's role in community mental health.

KEY TERMS

Burden of disease	Mental health
Community mental health	Mental health promotion
Community mental health center	Mental illness
	Neurosis
Community support programs	Psychosis
Deinstitutionalization	Serious and persistent mental illness (SPMI)
Disability-adjusted life year (DALY)	Serious mental illness (SMI)
Halfway house	Stigma
Insanity	

■ Teaching Strategies

CLASSROOM TEACHING STRATEGIES

1. Invite a community mental health professional (nurse) to class to speak about her or his role in preventive programs offered in the community. How does this role differ from the role of community health nurses who work with the general population? If this person is not a nurse, how does she or he collaborate with the community health nursing staff on community mental health issues?

2. Invite a counselor from the college health services to discuss the services offered to students at the three levels of prevention in regards to mental health issues and crisis intervention.

CLINICAL LABORATORY TEACHING STRATEGIES

1. Plan to have the clinical laboratory students attend at least one open 12-step program meeting, such as AA, NA, GA, or OA. During a clinical conference have the students share their experiences. Do the students feel these programs are effective? If so, why do they work?

2. As part of the clinical laboratory experience, have students observe or work in a community mental health center. They should observe or participate in group counseling sessions for clients or family members, if allowed by the staff and if they have completed their psychiatric nursing clinical laboratory experience. After all students have participated, discuss the dynamics of the counseling sessions as a therapeutic intervention for clients as well as family members during a clinical conference.

ACTIVITIES TO PROMOTE CRITICAL THINKING IN THE CLASSROOM

1. Discuss various suicide prevention programs at the primary level of prevention for people of different ages—teens, middle-aged individuals, the elderly. How will you measure the effectiveness of the intervention techniques?

2. Consider the cultural variations within your community. What groups are represented in the community? How does each view mental illness? What cultural practices do they use to treat mental illness? How does the medical community deal with these cultural differences when attempting to treat mental illness?

3. Discuss the variety of families you serve in the clinical laboratory setting. Which ones would benefit from mental health interventions at the primary level? Provide program suggestions and plan to implement at least one with a group of clients. An example might be a mothers-of-toddlers support group that meets for 6 weeks for an hour and is led by a small group of community health nursing students.

4. Discuss recent acts of violence occurring in local schools. Sources might be newspaper articles or personal experiences in the local community. Discuss how the situation was handled at the secondary level of prevention and what measures followed at the tertiary level of prevention. Does the class have any suggestions for improving the actions taken?

5. Facilitate a class discussion about depression and the elderly, especially among elderly men. Ask the students to share personal experiences of depression among older men in their family or among client families during their nursing education. What were some of the common themes expressed by these individuals? How have some of them dealt with the depression successfully? Are there any elderly men in the students' case load this semester? If so, how can they use what they know about depression and the elderly to promote the health of these inidividuals?

6. Have the students consider the group of clients they are serving in the community this term. Suggest that they select one category of stressors most experienced by these clients and search the Internet for information on effective inetrventions that address the issue. For example, a student may be serving several women who have experienced spousal abuse or have a history of sexual abuse as children; another student is working with elderly

women who are widows. Encourage the students to use the information to enhance their work with their clients.

■ Evaluation Strategies

MULTIPLE-CHOICE QUESTIONS

1. Dorothea Lynde Dix played an important role in the history of mental health. She is most known for:

   Humane treatment, health care, and social services for the mentally ill
   Dix worked in the 19th century to bring about reform that had been impemented in the U.S. and Europe by the end of the 1800s.

   Deistitutionalization of the mentally ill into community-based care settings
   This came about during the Reagan Administration in the early 1980s.

   Fighting to dispell the belief that the mentally ill were heretical agents of Satan
   Dix's work took place in the 1800s, and these beliefs were prevalent before the 13th century, leading to witch hunts.

   Founding the famous mental hospital in England, Saint Mary of Bethlehem
   This hospital was founded in 1450 and was commonly called "Bedlam." Dix's work occurred 400 years later.

2. When we look at the incidence and prevalence of mental disorders, the statistics for the United States include:

   Every year one out of five Americans experiences a diagnosable mental disorder.
   Each year 51 million Americans experience a diagnosable mental disorder.

   Each year half of the people with a diagnosed mental disorder are disabled by it.
   About 13%, or 6.5 million out of 51 million people, are disabled by an SMI.

   About 10% of the population of the United States suffers from bipolar disorder.
   Although a disruptive disorder, just 1% of the population suffer from it. However, 20% of those affected commit suicide.

   Attention-deficit/hyperativity disorder occurs in 1% of the school-aged population.
   The percentage is higher—3% to 5%—and it occurs four times more frequently in boys.

3. Specific risk factors influence the mentally ill population. Biological factors include:

Prenatal damage from exposure to alcohol, drugs, and tobacco
These are examples of biological factors influencing the mentally ill population.

Anxiety and emotional stress from economic hardship
These are examples of a sociocultural factor influencing the mentally ill population.

Psychological stress from neglect, abuse, or dysfunctional family life
These are examples of behavioral factors influencing the mentally ill population.

Climate and geography causing severe stresses due to extreme weather-related events
These are examples of environmental factors influencing the mentally ill population.

4. An example of a biomedical approach to meeting the needs of the mentally ill is:

Pharmacological therapy
This form of biomedical treatment includes one or more medications in the treatment regimen.

Behavior therapy
This form of psychotherapy aims to reduce or eliminate certain behaviors through concentrated, specific guidelines.

Group therapy
This form of psychotherapy uses the interaction of several clients sharing an interest in a common issue.

Insight-oriented therapy
This form of psychotherapy assists clients to improve their functioning through insight into themselves and their situation.

5. The community health mental health nurse should be aware of a variety of community mental health resources. One of the resources is a self-help group. This is:

A group of individuals who meet regularly to work on personal problems and issues
This describes a self-help group.

A group of multidisciplinary clinicians who travel to the scene of a crisis or critical event
This describes a mobile crisis team.

A publicly funded set of services designed to assist persons with mental illness
This describes community support programs.

A residential program for individuals with mental illness that includes supportive services
This describes a half-way house.

ESSAY QUESTIONS

1. An important role of the community mental health nurse is advocacy. Describe how this role can be carried out in the community and supply specific examples.

2. Select two of the following mental health programs or services and summarize what each offers: community support programs, mobile crisis teams, and self-help groups.

INDIVIDUAL OR GROUP PROJECTS

1. As a part of a group teaching project, contact an elementary school and offer to teach on the topic of mental health. In collaboration with the teacher, plan and implement age-appropriate activities that will promote mental health at the primary level of prevention. Such topics could include self-esteem, assertiveness, healthy expression of feelings, and so on.

2. Have a group of clinical laboratory students "adopt" a residential care facility (half-way house) for clients with mental illness. During the term the students can provide a variety of services: educational programs, social activities, and group discussions.

CHAPTER 35

Clients Living With Addiction

LEARNING OBJECTIVES

Upon mastery of this chapter, you should be able to:

- Define terms commonly used to describe addiction and addictive behaviors.

- Discuss the history and current incidence and prevalence of addiction in the U.S.

- Compare and contrast various theories on the etiology of addiction.

- Clarify your own assumptions and beliefs regarding clients living with addiction.

- Identify the *Healthy People 2010* goals for reducing addiction in the U.S.

- Discuss a variety of physical, psychosocial, and economic problems of clients, families, and communities struggling with addiction.

- Compare and contrast the preventive measures appropriate to clients addicted to alcohol, tobacco, other depressants, stimulants, and gambling.

- Describe the role of the nurse in caring for clients, families, and communities struggling with addiction.

KEY TERMS

Addiction	Substance abuse
Chemical dependence	Tolerance
Detoxification	Triggers
Polysubstance use and abuse	Withdrawal symptoms
Relapse	

■ Teaching Strategies

CLASSROOM TEACHING STRATEGIES

1. Ask for volunteers to share personal experiences dealing with a family member, friend, or acquaintance who abuses substances. Be sure the students share how being around the person made them feel and how the abuse affects the abuser's life and the people around her or him. You will need to ask for volunteers as many people feel uncomfortable sharing such information.

2. Brainstorm possible primary, secondary, and tertiary prevention strategies to use with clients experiencing addiction to _____ (choose a substance or activity for the sake of discussion).

CLINICAL LABORATORY TEACHING STRATEGIES

1. Have each clinical laboratory student attend an AA, NA, GA, or OA open meeting. During a clinical conference, have the students share their observations and impressions.

2. Have each clinical laboratory student become involved in providing services to groups of people at high risk for substance abuse. As a service to this aggregate, develop a teaching plan that focuses on primary prevention. For example, with a group of teens a nursing student might teach about not smoking and how to remain "cool," or with elementary or junior high school–aged children teach ways to say no by practicing various possible scenarios in which drugs, cigarettes, or alcohol might be involved.

ACTIVITIES TO PROMOTE CRITICAL THINKING IN THE CLASSROOM

1. Discuss whether prohibition was a viable way to stop the consumption of alcohol. Is this argument similar to the legalized abortion issue? Does making alcohol consumption or abortion illegal stop it from happening?

2. Offer these six questions to the class for discussion. All topics may take more than one class period to discuss as there will be many feelings shared about each one. If time is limited, allow just 10 or 15 minutes per question and choose three or four key questions.

3. Ask the students to share the Internet resources they found on local and regional substance abuse treatment programs. Discuss them in class. Suggest that a small group of students put them together as a resource file for the clinical laboratory.

■ Evaluation Strategies

MULTIPLE-CHOICE QUESTIONS

1. The history of addictive behavior in the U.S. and other countries includes the following fact:

Cocaine was popular for medicinal purposes in the U.S. in the 1800s.
Merck Pharmaceutical Company produced cocaine in the 1860s. Freud published a book titled On Coca in 1884. Cocaine was being used as a local anesthetic in eye surgery in the 1880s.

Opium is essentially a new drug to be abused; it was first used in the 1800s.
Opium has been used as early as 3000 BC in Sumeria and China. When it appeared in the United States in the 1700s, it was unrestricted and cheaper than alcohol, and people became addicted.

The Women's Christian Temperance Union was formed to decrease the use of opium and cocaine.
This organization was established to decrease the consumption of alcohol and cigarettes.

Alcoholics Anonymous (AA) was formed by two female physicians in 1975.
It was formed by two men, one of whom was a physician, 40 years earlier in 1935.

2. The three most prevalent drugs abused by adolescents include:

Alcohol, cigarettes, and marijuana
These are the three drugs most abused by adolescents.

Marijuana, cocaine, and opium
These are not the three drugs most abused by adolescents.

Cocaine, alcohol, and opium
These are not the three drugs most abused by adolescents.

Cigarettes, cocaine, and marijuana
These are not the three drugs most abused by adolescents.

3. The most used and abused drug among all age groups is:

Alcohol
51% of people use alcohol, and 7% to 10% abuse alcohol.

Marijuana
Alcohol is the most used and abused drug.
Cocaine
Alcohol is the most used and abused drug.

Opium
Alcohol is the most used and abused drug.

4. Chemical addiction is:

Determined to be an illness by scientific research conducted in the 20th century
This is the accepted belief, and the approach to those addicted is dependent on this.

A behavior that could be stopped if the person exercised willpower
Chemical addiction is a disease, and more intensive therapy is needed.

A choice, and therefore does not meet the criteria to classify it as a disease
Chemical addiction is a disease, and the addiction is not a choice; however, the first time used it was a choice.

Always accompanied by addiction to other substances and behaviors
Chemical addiction is a disease and may be the only addiction; however, people may have more than one addiction at a time—for example, smoking and gambling, drinking and gambling, or smoking and using marijuana.

5. The following actions constitute primary prevention efforts on the part of a community health nurse to reduce and or eliminate substance abuse:

Teaching teens about the genetic predisposition to alcohol addiction
This is an example of primary prevention—teaching prior to use/abuse.

Assessing a person entering an alcohol treatment program for the amount of use
This is an example of secondary prevention—the person is receiving treatment for the addiction.

Determining the readiness of an individual for treatment and choice of intervention
This is an example of secondary prevention—the person is being assessed for readiness to accept treatment for the addiction.

Planning a program that is designed to help individuals prevent drug use relapses
This is an example of tertiary prevention—the person is being helped to remain drug free after receiving treatment for the addiction.

ESSAY QUESTIONS

1. In 200 words or less, describe how it might feel to be the drug-free spouse of a woman addicted to drugs; you have two young children, ages 3 years and 10 months, and you must go to work every day to support your family.

2. You are the community health nurse providing services to the family in essay question 1. What services would you provide? When and whom would you visit? What teaching might you do? What community services would you recommend?

INDIVIDUAL OR GROUP PROJECTS

1. As a whole class or in smaller groups, plan a health fair for the junior high or high school–aged population in your clinical laboratory community. Focus the fair on addiction prevention. Invite community resources to sponsor booths and bring pamphlets and other materials. Collaborate with school administration and classroom teachers to make this a successful event. Include short teaching sessions, rewards for going to each booth, and door prizes. Use the school gymnasium or cafeteria and make arrangements for students to attend the fair during gym class, health class, or free periods.

2. Include work in a homeless shelter as part of the clinical laboratory experience. Students can participate in their health clinic activities, help cook and serve at mealtimes, or assist in a child care center (if the shelter has one) while interacting with the people staying there. In addition, in a small group or as an individual, organize an activity for the drop-ins or residents that is fun and educational—perhaps a game of Bingo in which they win food products or vouchers for clothing or another game in which correct answers to health questions win a food or clothing prize. This could be geared towards the children with the parents' help or for adults alone.

CHAPTER 36

Clients in Correctional Facilities

LEARNING OBJECTIVES

Upon mastery of this chapter, you should be able to:

- Define a variety of terms associated with correctional health care and correctional institutions.

- Describe the correctional culture and environment.

- Describe the history of correctional health care.

- Identify the key issues and challenges of correctional health care.

- List and describe at least four organizations associated with inmates of correctional facilities.

- Identify the communicable diseases and physical and mental health disorders commonly seen in correctional populations.

- Discuss the special areas of concern for nurses working with incarcerated women.

- Describe the role of the community health nurse while working with populations in correctional facilities.

KEY TERMS

Correctional facility	Maximum security
Felony	Minimum security
Forensics	Penitentiary
Inmates	Prison
Jail	Recidivism
Literacy	

■ Teaching Strategies

CLASSROOM TEACHING STRATEGIES

1. Invite a corrections nurse to speak to the class about her or his role in a corrections facility. Inquire into her or his working relationship with the guards and prisoners. Often the nurse walks a fine line between these two populations. How does this nurse manage that balance and still act as an advocate for the inmates? What are some of the major health problems that the incarcerated population exhibits? Are these problems different from correctional facilities in other parts of the country?

2. If possible, invite someone to class who has served time in a prison and inquire about her or his view of the health services in the facility. What particular stressors did this person experience while incarcerated? You may be able to find a speaker through a prison advocacy group, through clients in the clinical laboratory setting, or through connections with parole officers or the police department.

3. If possible, invite someone who has experienced a violent crime and explore his or her experiences during the arrest, trial, conviction, time served, and possibly the release or execution of the perpetrator. What services are available for victims of crimes and family members? What were some of the personal stressors this victim or family experienced? What would this victim or family suggest is the most important thing nurses should be aware of in regards to the experiences they shared?

CLINICAL LABORATORY TEACHING STRATEGIES

1. Plan to have the students spend some time in a corrections facility working with the nurses in the health services program. An especially receptive setting is a juvenile facility.

2. After the students have been providing care to all of the clients they will see during the term, inquire during a clinical conference how many of the clients or family members are or have been incarcerated. Are the students surprised by the numbers who have served or are serving a jail sentence? What were their crimes? Does knowing this information about clients alter how the students feel about caring for them?

ACTIVITIES TO PROMOTE CRITICAL THINKING IN THE CLASSROOM

1. Discuss the case scenario depicted in this activity. How would the class handle the situation? What issues are inherent in this case?

2. Discuss the case scenario depicted in this activity. How would the class handle the situation? What issues are inherent in this case?

3. Discuss the case scenario depicted in this activity with the class. Have the students work in small groups and give them different aspects of the case to work on. For example, if you divide the class into three groups, have one group respond to the various situations among the male population, another group identify the epidemiological triad, and the third group develop a plan that includes the three levels of prevention.

4. Have each student gather at least two websites that contain information about correctional nursing and particular problems in the incarcerated population. When all students have completed this, discuss their findings in class. Perhaps a student or small group of students will compile this information into one resource file for use by this class or the next.

■ Evaluation Strategies

MULTIPLE-CHOICE QUESTIONS

1. In the United States, including city and county jails and state and federal prisons, approximately how many people are detained each year?

Just under 2 million men and women
In 1999 there were 600,000 persons in city and county jails and 1.2 million in state and federal prisons.

One million men and very few women
In 1999 there were 600,000 persons in city and county jails and 1.2 million in state and federal prisons. Women represent about 8% to 10% of the incarcerated population, or about 140,000.

Ten million men and women
In 1999 there were 600,000 persons in city and county jails and 1.2 million in state and federal prisons.

Just over 5 million men and women
In 1999 there were 600,000 persons in city and county jails and 1.2 million in state and federal prisons.

2. African-American women are an over-represented minority in jails, prisons, and penitentiaries, and the following figures describe the numbers of these women:

They are less than 15% of the U.S. population but represent 52% of incarcerated women.
This is true, according to Human Rights Watch, 1996.

They are about 5% of the U.S. population but represent 25% of incarcerated women.
This is not true, according to Human Rights Watch, 1996; they are less than 15% of the U.S. population but represent 52% of incarcerated women.

They are less than 1% of the U.S. population but represent 10% of incarcerated women.
This is not true, according to Human Rights Watch, 1996; they are less than 15% of the U.S. population but represent 52% of incarcerated women.

They are about 20% of the U.S. population but represent 40% of incarcerated women.
This is not true, according to Human Rights Watch, 1996; they are less than 15% of the U.S. population but represent 52% of incarcerated women.

3. Historically, prisons were designed to be:

Punitive settings where prisoners forfeited all rights
This is true and, until 1929, prisons generally were administered on that basis.

Facilities where inmates were given correctional treatment
No treatment was designed or offered to correct an inmate's behavior.

Settings where people "worked off" their crimes
This was the intention of workhouses, an alternative to the prison setting in some communities about a century ago.

Safe havens from epidemics that spread across countries centuries ago
They were often beds of epidemics due to unsafe hygiene practices and close living conditions.

4. Several pieces of legislation have affected correctional health care. One document guarantees the right of prisoners to a safe and humane environment. This is found in:

The Eighth Amendment to the Constitution
This amendment guarantees the right of prisoners to a safe and humane environment.

The 1976 Supreme Court *Estelle v. Gamble* decision
This decision further clarified that correctional facilities could not deliberately show indifference to serious medical needs of prisoners.

The Violent Crime Control and Law Enforcement Act
This 1994 bill calls for mandatory sentencing for certain drug offenses.

The Prison Litigation Reform Act
This 1996 act requires correctional institutions to be responsible for the quality of health care delivered to individuals while incarcerated.

5. Correctional nurses function as community health nurses within correction facilities. Their roles include education, advocacy, and activist, and they act as a liaison between inmates and the community. A corrections nurse reports improprieties he observed while an inmate was being transported from the clinic to his cell block. This is an example of which of the following roles?

Advocacy
In this role the nurse speaks on behalf of the inmate to improve or correct a negative situation.

Education
In this role the nurse works to increase health knowledge among the prisoners.

Liaison
In this role the nurse acts as a bridge between the inmate and the outside community.

Activist
As an activist the nurse goes beyond the situation at hand and pursues changes that inhibit the continuation of negative actions. An activist has to be an advocate first.

ESSAY QUESTIONS

1. Respond to the following statement in 250 words or less: "They should lock child molesters up and throw away the key."

2. One of the key roles of the nurse working in corrections is that of advocate. Describe how you would advocate for women in a correctional facility. Include three specific actions you could take.

INDIVIDUAL OR GROUP PROJECTS

1. With a small group of peers, work with the health team members of a local juvenile correctional facility to plan a series of teaching sessions. The youth respond positively to well-developed and creative teaching plans presented by nurses who are comfortable in the setting and with the teaching topics. Topics of interest to them include appropriate expression of feelings, healthy relationships, human sexuality, keeping your body strong and healthy, and so on.

2. "Adopt" a unit or cell block in a local correctional facility and provide ongoing activities and services throughout the term, year, or for the length of the nursing program, if possible. Conduct small group health-related teaching sessions, participate in activities for social diversion such as arts and crafts or games (all must be cleared with the corrections staff as the first and foremost objective of the institution is security), and include something special for certain holidays.

CHAPTER 37

Clients in Home Health, Hospice, and Long-Term Care Settings

LEARNING OBJECTIVES

Upon mastery of this chapter, you should be able to:

- Describe the home care, hospice, and long-term care populations.

- Discuss standards and credentialing for home care, hospice, and long-term care nursing.

- Provide an overview of the evolution of home care, hospice, and long-term care nursing.

- Identify a variety of home care and long-term care agencies.

- Explain the roles and responsibilities of the various members of the home health, hospice, and long-term care team.

- Describe the reimbursement systems common to home health, hospice, and long-term care.

- Describe the role of the community health nurse in meeting the health care needs of the homebound population.

- Describe the role of the community health nurse in meeting the health care needs of the hospice family.

- Describe the role of the community health nurse in meeting the health care needs of clients in long-term care settings.

KEY TERMS

Assisted living	Informal caregivers
Durable medical equipment	Long-term care
Formal caregivers	Ombudsman
Home health care	Palliative care
Home health nursing	Respite
Homebound	Skilled nursing facility (SNF)
Homemaker agency	Skilled nursing services
Hospice	Terminally ill
Hospital-based agency	

■ Teaching Strategies

CLASSROOM TEACHING STRATEGIES

1. Ask the director of a home health agency to speak to the class about the services provided by her or his agency. Ask the guest to include assets she or he looks for in prospective nurses hired.

2. Conduct a seminar that compares the philosophy of a for-profit home health agency with that of a public health department in the community. Compare and contrast the roles and functions each serves in the community.

3. Invite a nursing administrator from a long-term care setting or hospice program to speak to the class and share the role of the registered nurse in her or his agency. What assets does the administrator look for in newly hired nurses?

CLINICAL LABORATORY TEACHING STRATEGIES

1. Have the students visit a private retirement village and compare the levels of satisfaction and the health care needs and services found in that setting with those of an elderly population living in their own homes or apartments among people of all ages. How do the people compare in the two situations?

2. Ask students to assess the community for service providers who provide home health care. They should find out what type of payment plan is required and what gaps in service exist.

3. Compare the process of dying in a hospital setting versus through the services of a hospice program— either the home care services or those of an inpatient hospice program. How do they differ? Which would you prefer your family members were a part of if they were dying?

ACTIVITIES TO PROMOTE CRITICAL THINKING IN THE CLASSROOM

1. Facilitate a general discussion about home health, hospice and long-term care nurses. Are their roles more alike or different? Why are they considered community health nurses?

2. Initiate a discussion about the rewards of hospice nursing. As a different way to participate in a discussion, play the "devil's advocate" and defend all parts of this type of nursing as students ask you challenging questions about working with the dying, or deny any benefits or rewards in this type of nursing as students share their own positive views.

3. Use the content of this activity to generate a general discussion about aging and housing choices. If students say they will stay in their home until they die, challenge them to consider who will do the yard work, cleaning, cooking, and so on—who will pay for these services? Do the students know about long-term care insurance, and would they buy such a premium?

4. Near the end of the term, after the students have had an opportunity to make shared visits with home health nurses, discuss their observations, levels of participation, and whether they would consider this type of nursing in the future.

5. Discuss the findings from the students' exploration of hospice programs in the region. Encourage a student to compile the findings to create a hospice resource file for future use by students in community health nursing or to be given to the staff of the clinical laboratory agency.

■ Evaluation Strategies

MULTIPLE-CHOICE QUESTIONS

1. When you work with informal caregivers as a home care or hospice nurse, you should:

   Focus on caretaker abilities, not their limitations
   Keep a positive attitude that is focused on abilities, not limitations, of the caregivers.

   Include only the spouse or significant other in the plan
   Include all family members and caregivers in the plan.

   Visit frequently to manage and maintain equipment
   Teach family members and caregivers how to manage and maintain equipment.

   Choose what you feel is the most important thing to teach first
   Choose an area to teach first that the client or caretaker is motivated to learn, to help keep frustration low.

2. The coordinator of care in home care is the:

   Registered nurse
   The registered nurse is considered the coordinator of care.

   Social worker
   The social worker is another clinical staff member but is not the coordinator of care.

   Physician
   The physician directs the skilled care to clients by agreeing (signing the nurse-generated paperwork) with the plan of care established by the registered nurse who coordinates the care.

   Dietician
   The dietician is another clinical staff member but is not the coordinator of care.

3. The philosophy of hospice care includes:

   Holistic and family-centered care to terminally ill clients
   This is the philosopy of hospice care.

   The right to die and encourages euthanasia
   Hospice care is delivered to terminally ill people with the recognition that death is a human experience, but euthanasia is not part of the care.

   Working with people in their last year of life
   Hospice care can be initiated after a physician has declared that a person has 6 months or less to live.

   Weaving hospice concepts around curative treatment
   Hospice care is initiated in the final phase of a person's illness when he or she is not receiving curative treatment.

4. One of the criteria for receiving Medicare-reimbursed home care is that the client is:

   Homebound
   This is a requirement and means the person can only leave the home with difficulty and only for medical appointments or adult day care.

   Visited by a homemaker
   Medicare requires that the recipient of reimbursible services need skilled services. The services of a homemaker are not considered a skilled service and are not a requirement for receiving services.

   A veteran
   There are no requirements that the client be associated with the military, either now or in the past.

Terminally ill

This is required to receive hospice services reimbursed by Medicare but not home health care—the person would just require skilled services.

5. Which of the following definitions best describes an assisted living arrangement?

A setting designed to provide housing, personalized supportive services, and health care based on need for those who require help with ativities of daily living

This best describes an assisted lving arrangement.

A setting designed to meet the caregiving needs of frail individuals who need long-term rehabilitative, recuperative, or custodial care that includes skilled procedures and equipment

This describes a skilled nursing facility.

A philosophy of care that focuses on a holistic and family-centered approach to care and living until one dies, with death accepted as a human experience

This describes the philosophy of hospice.

The skilled observation and assessment, teaching, and performance of procedures that require nursing judgment

This describes skilled nursing services and does not describe an assisted living choice.

ESSAY QUESTIONS

1. In your own words, explain the difference between home health care service clients and community health nursing service clients.

2. How do you envision health care in the year 2025 (probably a time when you will be at the peak of your years of practice)? Where will health care be provided? Who will use the hospitals in 2025? Will technology change? Will home care, long-term care, and hospice care services change? Will they increase or decrease?

INDIVIDUAL OR GROUP PROJECTS

1. Ask the director of a home health agency to allow you to participate in a chart audit on some clients. How does it differ from chart audits on hospitalized clients? Share this experience with classmates, if all students were not involved. If all students were involved, compare and contrast ageny protocol.

2. If a group of students made home visits to home health care clients, share information about clients visited with common diagnoses (diabetes, CHF, CVA, etc.). Discuss how the agencies are managing client care. What supports do the clients have? How different is the support each client receives from families and friends? What makes the difference in their ability to manage well? How can the home care nurse make a difference in clients' response to illness and follow-up care?